Why We Are

WIRED TO WORRY

And How Neuroscience
Will Help You Fix it

Stop Stressing, Reduce Anxiety, <u>Feel</u> Happy — Finally!

by Sharie Spironhi

Worry-Go-Round™ Sharie Spironhi

Publisher: Sharie Spironhi

Book Design and Layout: Sharie Spironhi

Cover Design: Sharie Spironhi

Copy Editing: Carol Grampp

Inside and Cover Photos: Dollar Photo Club

Back Cover Photo of Author: ZeeZee Shots Photography

ISBN-13: 978-1508616276

ISBN-10: 1508616272

Contact Information: www.SharieSpironhi.com

FOR MOM & DAD. THANKS FOR EVERYTHING.

If you need an extra workbook or want a recording of the Guided Meditations click here or go to my website www.shariespironhi.com

To get the most out of this book you need to utilize the workbook!

CONTENTS

Before you begin your journey let me welcome you!
I applaud your efforts to improve your life.
You are going to learn things you never knew
before and if you put them to use your life is
going to change drastically for the better.
Join our facebook group—
www.facebook.com/groups/GetOffYourWorryGoRound/
There you can have discussions
and compare experiences with other readers.
Enjoy your journey!

INTRODUCTION

It's been a long day, you are exhausted and hope to be asleep before your head even hits the pillow. Instead just as you get comfortable a thought makes its was into your mind. And before you know it you are tossing, turning, and suddenly uncomfortable as emotions of anger, worry, and frustration consume you. What the hell just happened?

Day in and day out the same presumptuous fears, hypothetical "what ifs" concerns and worries get recycled from the previous day to rob us of peace. What makes this even more bizarre is that we always seem to persevere, no matter what life throws at us, and yet each day we react as though we are about to be crushed by the "next thing". It is because evolution has dropped the ball on us. Literally, right on our head. It still thinks we are in the jungle fighting tigers for our life and strangers for our food. It has no idea we can now get our breakfast by simply handing a stranger some money in exchange for a bag of food, an effort that requires nothing more than reaching a hand out of the car window. Why our reptilian brain didn't evolve right along with our ability to think, and reason, is still a mystery, but thankfully we don't have to be under its power anymore. Controlling our stress is not a matter of waiting until the planets line up and put us into better circumstances although that is what most people seem to believe.

Seventy-seven percent of the US population suffers from physical symptoms related to stress. Stress is our reaction to disappointments and problems both real and imagined. It originates from within us, so it is there that we have to begin to fix it and thankfully science is offering us the tools to do just that.

We are funny creatures; some of us just want to know what to do to change while others need to know why we are broken to begin with. I am of the latter group, and I wrote this book for others who want to know how we got here. When I find I have lost my way in any area, it has always served me best to find out how I got lost to begin with. This also correlates well with my innate desire to teach others and explain things. So here we go, people of the *why*.

Happiness evades you because your brain does not care about being happy. It is not wired to seek happiness and does not even place it on your priority list. Of course, you may be thinking, "Wait a minute—I absolutely care about being happy; it's why I bought this damn book." But that is your mind talking, not your brain, and your mind and brain are not the same. Your mind is the consciousness that resides within your brain. The part of you that chases happiness in all it's forms. However, your brain's number-one job for the past ten thousand years, has been your survival, and to this day its primary goal remains keeping you alive at any cost, even if that cost is your happiness. How it does this is by obsessively looking for danger, which to your brain is anything at all that might

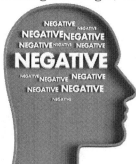

threaten your life in five areas: **love, money, status, health, and security.** Anything that can threaten these areas can threaten your life as far as your brain is concerned. This has turned your brain into a magnet for problems both real and imagined. It is that constant echo of "Careful, oh no, watch out!" Ringing in your ears. That's its job—your survival. It cares about danger, not about your state of unhappiness.

In the past decade, science has uncovered many exciting new details about how the brain works. Technology is allowing us a deeper look into the human mind, helping us to understand more clearly why it is on constant high alert for danger, and why it tends to ignore all of the everyday positive things in our lives. Uplifting experiences, such as hugs, "I love you's," compliments, or a sharing of hearts, are trivial to your brain because let's face it, a hug won't help you fight a tiger off. This once powerful tool for survival could now be costing us our life, through physical illness and emotional breakdowns.

In this book, I will explain how your brain uses this negative bias to protect you physically, emotionally, and even socially—but leaves you sad, frustrated, exasperated, emotional, and feeling defeated in the process. You will learn why your reactions are overblown, why you do things you know are bad for you, and why you say things you wish you didn't. You will be amazed as you see how this outdated brain program has even shaped our culture into one that is obsessed with fame, fortune and status.

However, knowing the "whys" is only half the story; my goal is to bridge the gap between knowing *why* you do things and understanding *how* you can do them differently. This book will offer proven steps and techniques that will allow you to begin controlling your own moods and behavior. Striving to keep this book simple yet interesting, I will often use basic metaphors common to everyday life, so if you are from the scientific arena, please don't send me an angry e-mail for oversimplifying.

There are four names I will use throughout this book that may be new to you. Three are key neurochemicals—**dopamine**, **oxytocin**, and **serotonin**—while the other one refers to an area in your brain called the **amygdala**. These are the driving force behind all of your behaviors related to food, sexual preferences, social contact, the people you keep close, and the groups you associate with.

You will learn a blend of techniques and practices that will give you an eye-opening awareness that produces a huge shift in your mood toward real happiness. I will be implementing the latest neuroscience discoveries and my own experiences into practices that you can begin right away so that you will feel happier, less stressed, and less anxious in only two to four weeks.

The brilliant neuroscientists, psychologists, and neurobiologists of the past two decades have been paving the way for a better understanding of human behavior, many building on each other's discoveries. I do not have that scientific background. I began my journey into this arena in the early '80s, working in the addiction field at twenty-two years of age. I studied pharmacology because, back then, it offered the most insight on how drugs damaged the brains of addicts who now in sobriety were struggling to control their moods.

As the saying goes, "We love to teach what we want to learn"; Through my teens and 20's I had been struggling to control my own exaggerated moods. I read every medical book and all the research I could get my hands on, trying to parse out what light they could shed on my own struggle.

I worked in the addiction field for five years, as a producer of the David Toma show on WOR and later on as the director of the David Toma Center in Tecate, Mexico, a rehabilitation center for drugs and alcohol. Living in Mexico and spearheading the opening of this center created immense pressure. I came home after six months severely burned out and with my moods all over the place. When I finally went to a doctor, I was diagnosed as a rapid cycling manic depressive with mixed states, known these days as bi-polar disorder. Bipolar disorder is a complex disorder that comes from a combination of genetic and non-genetic factors. The mood episodes associated with it involve clinical depression or mania (extreme elation and high energy) with periods of normal mood and energy in between episodes. My periods of feeling normal were very short lived no more than 2-3 months at a time. It was 1990, and my life came to a crashing halt. I was twenty-seven years old; until then, I had been doing very well in my field. To be labeled mentally ill while I was working in the mental health field was a crushing blow. The abridged version is that I spent the next five and a half years in and out of hospitals, with stays as long as six weeks. Then in 1996, I had an experience that literally rewired my brain in four nights, leaving me free of all bi-polar symptoms.

Up until recently science could not speculate on what might have occurred in my brain to make such a drastic change over night. (This is also referred to as a "spontaneous healing") But more recently some discoveries have emerged from the world of neuroscience that provided the framework for understanding how something like that can take place in the brain. The biggest of those discoveries is that the human brain is changing all the time. It can be rewired, altered, shaped, and made to adapt. For the last 19 years I have been 100 percent free from any bipolar symptoms.

I have had my share of daily ups and downs with stress levels high enough to light up NYC. But two years ago I began to wonder if there was a way to retrain my brain to think differently if it could change so drastically in 4 nights. Well there was.

Over the past five years, we have learned more about the human brain than we had in the previous 50 years. Thanks to these brilliant discoveries, a path has finally been lit to take us on a wonderful journey into that mysterious three-pound mass on our shoulders. Although it is the most complex frontier in our universe, and we have only taken baby steps, we do have an understanding now that can provide us with some degree of control to obtain the kind of emotional life we have always wanted.

I wrote this book to give you the tools you need to do just that. I will describe some very complex communication within your brain, using simplistic descriptions; however, if you want more of the scientific underpinnings, author and neuropsychologist Rick Hansen has done a great job of writing two very in-depth books (Hardwiring Happiness and Stress Proof Your Brain) that were indispensable in creating this book.

I have read my share of self-help books, and, although motivating and insightful, most tell you only what you do wrong and why but not what you should do differently or how to do so, in detailed steps. In this book you will learn tangible, measurable steps that can change your life, and that is what sets this book apart. Step by step, thought by thought, and belief by belief, I will take you deeper into your thinking and behavior so that you can truly understand for the first time what is driving your actions. This information is easy to understand and apply even without attending one of my workshops. I use tangible examples in everyday life, with metaphors and explanations of human behavior that will help you learn new conscious ways of thinking so that you will see very fast results. This is a journey; enjoy it. Chapter 2 is where you will learn details about your three key neurochemicals; let that info sink in throughout the book rather than overwhelming yourself by trying to memorize them. Trust me; by the end of the book, you will know them. You will find yourself referring back to this information as you see for the first time the real reasons behind your behavior and that of those around you. The first five chapters will take you on a very interesting journey into the workings of your brain and how your behavior has evolved to make you who you are. Be patient as you digest some new things; these will be your foundation as you come to understand your behavior better than ever before.

Stress and worry are the culprits robbing you of a happy life. Up until now it has not been your fault but rather your *default*. But you are responsible for what you know. So if you like being miserable, anxious and feeling like a victim then don't read any further, because once you do you will have no more excuses. Here you will have all the control you need to dissolve your stress. Maybe you have been promised this before, but now someone will teach you where that control has been hiding and how to use it.

If you can answer "yes" to this stress test below, then rest assured that you have bought the right book.
Do you find yourself swearing whenever you spill or drop something?
Do you curse regularly at other drivers?
Does your baseline mood hover between 1and 6 most days?
Do small, mundane tasks annoy you, more than they should?
Do you tell people off in your head after the altercation is over?
Do you live for your weekends and vacations, just tolerating the days in between?
Do people ever tell you, "You need to calm down"?
Is your health suffering from stress?
Do you find it difficult to maintain your vacation "calm" once back home?

Come step behind the veil and see what has been pulling your strings.

Even if you don't feel overly stressed, don't think for a moment that you aren't at risk for health problems. The chemicals at play in your body are wreaking havoc with many of your systems; over time, that can do long-term damage. No amount of stress is OK on a long-term basis. Review the list below and see what symptom you experience now or have experienced this past year. This information has to factor into your commitment to making these changes.

Physical Health Consequences:

• Weakened immune system

• Digestive problems

• Decreased reproductive hormones

• Heart problems

If you have 3 or more symptoms you MUST to retrain your brain or suffer physical consequences.

Mental Health Consequences

• Lowers mood and increases pessimistic outlook

• Increases anxiety and irritability

• Increases learned helplessness/victim mentality

• Increases social withdrawal

• Weakens enthusiasm and motivation

• Increases tendency to overreact

• Causes forgetfulness

1

How Science Is Picking Up
Where Evolution Left Off

Imagine you are driving down a barren road when your car suddenly dies just as you pass a lone gas station. You know how to drive your car, but you never learned how it works because you didn't think you needed to. You coast into the station because you know you are supposed to put some kind of gas into the tank, and you assume that must be what it needs. There is a red light lit up on the dash, but because you have no idea what it means, you ignore it, put diesel fuel in your little sports car, and speed away until your car makes weird noises and stops dead, this time in the middle of nowhere. Hard to believe anyone would drive around with little to no understanding of their car's basic functioning. Makes you wonder who let them do that; didn't they want to know more about their vehicle? Sad to say, this is the way most people treat that three-pound mass above their neck. We know basically how it works, and to keep it running, we simply let it feed on any thoughts, images or emotions it wants, not to mention disregarding its need for sleep and nutrition. We walk around oblivious to the signs that it is in trouble until it is too late.

We perceive our moods as something mysterious, and believe if we can just figure out the magic recipe of behaviors, diet, and sleep, we will find happiness. Well, that is like getting into your car, putting the radio on, and expecting to keep the same station on for three hundred miles! That signal will pick up other frequencies, drop out completely, and pull in annoying static. Somehow, we just assume being happy should come naturally if we do the right things—but nothing could be further from the truth. It is time that human beings learn the fundamentals of how the human brain, the most sophisticated machine in the universe, works. We don't have to get too technical or be overwhelmed with a huge vocabulary, but it would be nice to at least know how to use our own brain to be a happier person. Sure, there may be a few terms in this book that you have not heard before, but that is part of learning something new. You had no idea what an IPad or GPS was fifteen years ago, but you know them now and understand how they work. It is no more logical to ignore new discoveries about the brain than to ignore new technology and expect to stay current with the world. We spend more time in a given year learning about our new smart phone than we ever do about our own brain. Well, it's time. What you have in your hand is a book that will teach you a few fundamentals about your brain that will change your life. No more living on autopilot, guessing at why you are in a good mood or assuming why you are in a bad one. You are going to learn how to make conscious decisions that will control the performance of your brain and mind. This stuff is as basic as understanding why you turn your lights off and take your keys with you when you exit your vehicle.

Don't you want to be happy and have less static in your life? Most of us are so stressed by our jobs and responsibilities that we live for our weekends and vacations and hate the days in between.

We waste precious energy trying to manage the awful feelings and physical effects of stress. It is why we overeat, crave comfort foods, drink too much, sleep too much or not enough, take risks, sleep with people we don't know, and beg our doctor for prescriptions to stop the pain. Living in this state causes all kinds of physical and mental illnesses, and it wreaks havoc with our relationships. Did you know surveys have shown that many healthy individuals are less happy than cancer patients and people in wheelchairs? In the absence of these difficulties, we should be waking up every morning singing to Pharrell Williams's song "Because I'm Happy." Americans spend almost $700 million per year on self-help books. The topics vary from becoming a better communicator, parent, or spouse to losing weight. Categorically, we can define our intention to feel better, act better, or be better together as the common goal. Therefore reducing our stress level in some way and becoming happier.

Our misery starts with a false belief that our natural emotional state is *supposed to be one of happiness*, with happiness defined as a sense of well-being and contentment. Most of us believe that if all of life's problems just left us alone, we would be happy. We believe it is only because we are disrupted by the everyday pressures of life that we are stressed out. Therefore, we spend most of our time trying to fix the "next thing" in an effort to find some peace. When we believe this, we could not be more mistaken. Science has now revealed that it is the opposite. **Being happy is not our default state of mind!** What is our natural default state? After about four years of age, our default state starts to evolve into one of **shyness, insecurities, caution, and defensiveness.** Genuine happiness can only be found on the inside because that is where our perception of problems start. Otherwise, most of our efforts toward self improvement are akin to giving our car a new paint job instead of a tune-up.

Our brain evolved over thousands of years to serve one goal, and that was to keep us alive. The problem is, it is still doing that job the same way it did back then: by being **obsessed with every possible negative outcome**. We come hardwired to be prepared for the worst-case scenario, and this negative focus has all of us walking on eggshells, waiting for the crap to hit the fan 24/7. It never allows us to relax or be too happy, and it even downplays good events with the proverbial, "Yeah, but..." or "What if?"

One hundred percent of all your misery or lack of joy and happiness is due to your brain's five basic fears. These control 90 percent of your brain's thoughts; loss of **love, money, status, health**, and **security**. Did you catch the key word here? Fear, an extreme emotion over what *might* happen! We live in fear of losing any of these five things even when we have an ample supply of them. We all know that rich guy who is always saying he's broke. The strategy for most of us has been to try to accumulate more love, money, status, health, and security so that we can be happy. Some of us even try to reject comfort and riches in the hopes that doing so will free us from this chase. However, the problem with trying to accumulate more and more is that the brain will never, ever tell us that we have enough! Never. This is the harsh reality that smacks most rich and famous people in the face, causing them to spin out of control. After they travel down this illusionary road for the promise of bliss, they discover that their brain is still not satisfied and continues to torture them with the fear of loss... which, to the brain, means loss of life. This is all part of our survival instinct; it is hardwired into the most primitive area of the human brain, not a switch we can just turn off. In essence, the brain is obsessed with chasing misery/problems both real and imagined in every area of our life—present, future, and past—in an effort to preserve love, money, status, health, and security. To your brain anything at all that could or might even graze those areas is reason to panic.

Until you understand how this happens, happiness, will **always** be outside your grasp. Today, if you can commit to some long-overdue rudimentary understanding of your brain, you will be on your way to finding the true happiness you deserve.

Julie came to me referred by a friend. She said, "I have a good life, but I worry that it will all end in some sort of crisis like I see in many of my friends' lives." She felt guilty for all of her blessings. Julie had become convinced that her feelings of fear were attached to some sort of future reality. How could they not be? Would anyone feel this way for no reason? There had to be impending doom. It took Julie only three weeks to put some understanding about her brain into practice and be able with absolute confidence to dismiss her feelings of guilt and worry as a result of her outdated warning system or her panic button, After three weeks, she wrote, "I can't believe the difference it makes to know where these negative thoughts come from! I was able to distance myself instantly, just as I would ignore a false alarm."

The Proverbial "Panic Button"

So which part of your brain actually sounds this alarm warning you of impending doom? It is a small, almond-sized area in your brain that evolved over thousands of years called the amygdala, also known

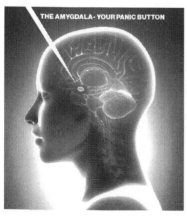

THE AMYGDALA - YOUR PANIC BUTTON

as your lizard brain. Pronounced, **ah-mig-da-la**. This part of the brain has been around forever, and every animal has it. The amygdala is no bigger than your fingernail, but it is the hub or control center for your emotions and determines what emotions to trigger, from elation to temper tantrums and worrying yourself sick. It is the switch for FIGHT or FLIGHT. It also does several other jobs, so unfortunately you can't just cut it out and go on your merry way. It helps you determine whether the face you are looking at is sad or happy, motivates you to find food when you are hungry, and helps you decide whether Eggplant Parmesan or a big steak will put a smile on your face. This little almond-shaped area helps you understand and process emotion both in you and around you. People who have been exposed to any kind of childhood trauma are likely to have a larger amygdala, with thicker connectivity to the areas around it, making it even more prone to emotional outbursts.

Something no bigger than your fingernail is responsible for all of this. You may hear some call it your lizard brain because it is in the oldest area of your brain, the part called the reptilian brain. These are all terms used to make it easy for you to remember it. However, the focus of this book is its role as your ALARM BELL. This personal warning system alerts you to problems real or imagined by making you feel horrible, by triggering stress-related hormones, such as cortisol (a hormone that, in excess is bad for your heart but good for adding belly fat—YUK!) and adrenaline. These hormones' job is to bring you to a heightened state of UH-OH or OH CRAP! Along with sensations of muscle tension, anxiousness, sweaty palms, heavy breathing, and rapid heartbeat. That is your brain's way of telling you to STOP, doing whatever it is you are doing!

For thousands of years, our amygdala functioned very well at keeping us alive in the wild by sending waves of these stress hormones such as adrenaline, cortisol, and epinephrine through our bodies as soon as we saw a lion in the bushes or a dangerous snake. It did that so we would do one thing... run like hell. Not worry, evaluate, or analyze it.

Back then, people's lives were in constant jeopardy, either from physical harm or from becoming a social outcast. Ten thousand years ago, if a woman's mate seemed unhappy with her, the woman's alarm bells would scream because if the man left, her family would have no food or protection and her offspring would die. The same happened when people were shunned by the other members of their tribe, causing them to become outcasts. That was a death sentence within hours. So it was not only the lion in the bushes but also the treatment they received from their inner social circle that meant life or death.

Now here you are today with a brain that is still interpreting any problem as a life-threatening situation! Your superior annoyed with you, a fight with your spouse, car trouble making you late for a meeting, or your in-laws coming for a two-week stay—all of these are often interpreted as life threatening as far as this little amygdala is concerned. It focuses on what will kill you—not on what keeps you happy—and therefore, so do you.

OUR OUTDATED BRAIN

10,000 YEAR OLD DANGERS	MODERN DAY PROBLEMS
SNAKES	TRAFFIC
TRIBAL OUTCAST	BOSS ANGRY
PARTNER ANGRY	CAR TROUBLE
LION/TIGERS	FINANCIAL STRESS
LACK OF FOOD	WORKLOAD
HUMAN ATTACK	SNIPPY COWORKER

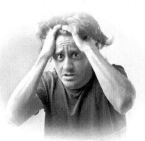

YOUR AMYGDALA THINKS THIS ALL COULD MEAN DEATH!

Although 90 percent of our problems in the twenty-first century are not life threatening, they trigger our amygdala. We need to reprogram the brain so that it doesn't hit this panic button simply because we received one hundred e-mails or because someone decided to do forty miles per hour in the fast lane. The human brain doesn't know that the coworker who gets snippy with us isn't life threatening. It senses a violation and sounds the alarm so that we come out swinging. Just knowing that we won't die from a dirty look is not enough to stop the alarm bell from telling us to prepare to pounce. We all see people overreacting to the slightest irritation—fights breaking out at sporting events, road rage, and so on—and we all know a hothead. The problem with employing common sense during these events is that this much older area of the brain responsible for emotion does not understand words and thoughts because it does not process language. It sees images and then judges, according to our past experiences, whether they are good for us, dangerous, or simply threaten any of those five areas I mentioned earlier. Once the brain sounds the siren, telling ourselves to calm down is pointless.

Like a gladiator jumping over a wall into the middle of a battle, that uneducated, ancient part of your brain has the final say regarding what you need to do to survive. Simply trying to think your way out of a panic will not help. Once the amygdala releases those fight-or-flight hormones into your system, it is all systems go! Have you ever tried telling someone who was yelling to calm down? A lot of good that did, right?

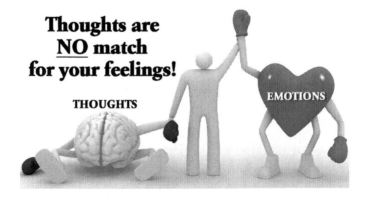

Thoughts are NO match for your feelings!

THOUGHTS   EMOTIONS

How long does it take for your amygdala to have your head spinning? Less than a second. For my women readers of a certain age, if you have ever had hot flashes, you can verify that they seem to come out of nowhere, very quickly, without provocation. Actually, hot flashes are due to a thought that just triggered a fear or concern, and it happens even when you are sleeping. You never noticed it because even a small concern causes your amygdala to react. While these chemicals are in play, you will feel very justified as you yell or have a tantrum, but when they dissipate, you wonder, "Why did I react like that and get upset over something so trivial?" You did it because your brain thought your life was in danger, and in the blink of an eye, you reacted instinctively.

In a social context, people with similar fears and frustrations will feel validated as they join together in groups, gangs, or cults. When the dreaded "group mentality" kicks in, a dangerous momentum can take place.

Your brain likes to be in agreement with others because staying with the crowd thousands of years ago gave you protection. Have you noticed that when you have a disagreement with someone, each of you is in defense mode? Your brain reacts as though the physical you—and not just your opinion—are in danger!

In this context, people may even join gangs or other groups

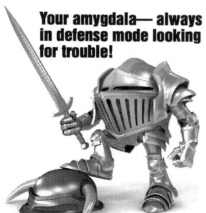

Your amygdala— always in defense mode looking for trouble!

with which they have very little in common other than their outrage, yet that one common factor can result in them taking violent political positions or engaging in all out war. All of the violence in the world can be traced back to an amygdala that screams, "**Kill or be killed!**"

Such situations are horribly dangerous because as we band together for a cause that may or may not be good, all reason and reality can slip away—leaving room only to validate what we want to believe. There are beliefs buried deep in our subconscious that we don't even know exist, yet they steer our actions. Our evolutionary instincts have left us blind to this behavior. For example the degree to which we align with and commit ourselves to a group or cause is the degree to which we see only what they are seeing. I don't really think we need to be told this however, we always think it the "others" who see only what they want. Like it or not it is us too. We don't mean to, it's not like we see the opposing facts and decide to ignore them, rather our brain only let's us see what is "best" for us. This is why the Middle East will never have peace and republicans and democrats will never understand how the opposing party can "see it " that way. Evolution has taught us that staying with "our group" is the best way to stay safe. Repeated studies have shown that we humans see only what we want to see, and hear only what we want to hear. This is why lawyers pick a jury according to what beliefs they hold, because they know they can sway them. The facts don't matter. A really good point to remember next time you are in argument. No one is immune to this. Hold your opinions lightly. As far as evolution is concerned, being objective and making our own decisions often is not in our best interest, so the brain always steers us toward going along with "our" crowd. Only an extremely self-aware person who has no ego will have a shot to evaluate something from a purely objective stance, regardless of what others think.

We do not easily change our perception of ourselves, others, or life. When we are unhappy we cling to our frustration/anger/misery much the same way a child clings to their security blanket. Doing so validates our years of pain, complaining and believing that life won't cut us a break. What if we just woke up happy one day and never worried again? Believe it or not, that can be a scary notion at first. After all, what would everyone think if we were suddenly happier for no real reason while in the same circumstances? Would our friends and family look at us and think we had been nothing but drama queens all this time? Probably not but they might champion our determination and validate our strength and tenacity for being able to be happy in spite of our difficulties and problems. They might even ask how we did it and want us to help them.

We all have genuine situations to deal with but at those times when your brain pushes the panic button over something small, I can assure you there is something else going on in your mind, and probably something unrelated. At the early stage of getting upset, you generally have an inaccurate perception of what is angering you. Underlying thoughts and memories from the past often attach themselves to the things happening in the present, causing you to overreact. You may be ruminating on something upsetting that took place yesterday when you suddenly spill something and let out a stream of expletives. All the while, you are completely unaware of what really triggered your outburst.

The core of this book will teach you how to separate an upsetting event from your ongoing undercurrent of worrisome thoughts. Only then will you be able to figure out what you are *really* feeling, and therefore how to feel better. Because that's your brain, a never-ending stream of what *ifs* and *worry* about how life did or will go wrong. Welcome to the *Worry-Go-Round*™

Worry-Go-Round™—*The time you waste going in circles rehashing the same fears, concerns and memories you had yesterday with no change. — Painted horses optional.*

The average person has between 32 and 48 thoughts per minute, according to the Laboratory of Neuro Imaging at the University of Southern California and the National Science Foundation. That can add up to a total of 70,000 thoughts per day! Several studies have also shown that 80 percent of those thoughts are negative, and 90 percent of which are similar to the ones you had the day before!

Feeling Happy Is a Learned Skill

The only way to overcome thoughts is with feelings. Thoughts are no match for feelings! You can't even calm yourself down; at times it can feel as though you are possessed. Right?

Feelings are to thoughts what water is to a flame. **We can't talk our way out of emotional pain; we have to feel our way out.** You can't be happy. Happy is not something you become. *You have to feel happy.* Until you learn how to *feel* happiness all around you, the majority of those negative seventy thousand thoughts per day will win out. If you were to try—and millions do every day—to just change your thoughts, how effective would you be even if you managed to fit in 10,000 positive thoughts among say, 50,000?

Saying you want to be happy is like saying you want to be rich. To accomplish either one takes understanding and learning beyond what you can figure out from reading books or magazines. You won't become rich just by avoiding financial losses; you have to actually make money at some point. Similarly, you will never become happy just by protecting those five areas of loss. You have to *accumulate feelings of happiness.* The first step toward feeling better is to teach your mind to begin focusing on all the good facts around you exactly the way it has been focusing on the negative. Before you dismiss this concept remember I explained that we only see what we want to see. Until you understand some concepts your reality is distorted, meaning two things. You think you *do see* all the good and it pales in comparison to your problems or you don't think you have much good around you. Trust me both are wrong.

Thus far, your brain is programmed to overlook most good things except those that relate to preserving your life, so that is the first thing we are going to change. This may seem trite or silly. Most people think they are aware of all the good around them. We count our blessings, as they say. However, acknowledging that something is good is very different from taking ten to twenty seconds to dwell on it so you can *feel* it on an emotional level. A study published in 2010 reported that when experiencing positive events, focusing attention on the present moment and engaging in positive rumination promotes a sense of well-being. Conversely, being *distracted* while *having* a good experience *lowers* the sense of well-being. How many times have you taken a few seconds to replay a compliment over in your mind until you actually felt happy about it? Probably never. Have you ever taken ten seconds to replay a hug from your loved one and really feel touched by the love? This is where everything changes! Feeling the good around you will permeate the emotional area in your brain where *words cannot reach*. **You can't talk your way into a good mood; you must feel your way.** You will learn to deliberately seek and hold onto the positive things around you, allowing these observations to become amazing feelings that sink into your whole being. I remember telling someone that it is possible to feel happy in mere seconds, but before I could explain it, the person blurted out, "OK, make me happy right now." We were standing in line at a store, but I figured it would pass the time. I asked her if she had a pet or child, and she said she had a beautiful golden retriever. She closed her eyes, and I told her to pretend she was on the floor with him after being out all day, and he was kissing her and welcoming her back home. In only eight seconds, a smile spread across her face. She opened her eyes, and I asked, "So do you feel happier than you did a few seconds ago?" She said, "Yeah! I can't wait to be home. I feel so much love for my dog right now!" She said she felt love, warmth, and a sense of everything being OK regardless of the issues in her life. She wasn't dismissing those issues, but for a moment, she stopped worrying about them.

This practice is quick even by today's standards; all it takes is waiting 10 to 20 seconds for a positive feeling to sink in. Then, like magic, your brain will turn that feeling into a memory, giving you something to feel good about. You do this now all day long by ruminating on mere potential problems and then feeling like your life is a potential powder keg. Why? Because reality and fiction are irrelevant to the brain it can't tell the difference which is why you get upset way before stuff actually happens.

Take twenty seconds right now to envision a person or pet showering you with love; Yes that means you. Put the book down. Really feel the love filling you. Did you feel the emotional lift? Now imagine carrying that feeling around most of the day. Can you picture how different you would feel if you did this regularly?

Harnessing the power of your imagination can change your life. It is the tool you will use throughout this book to transport you to momentary feelings of contentment, peacefulness, and well-being. If it seems silly to use your imagination or to waste ten seconds waiting to have a good feeling about something, consider this: most of us cherish the thousands of hours we spend watching movies and TV shows just so we can feel a whole host of emotions. We love our emotions, and we seem to like them even more when we can feel them without having to go through the actual trials that the actors portray.

If you have ever had a really good dream about your boss, coworker, or just some acquaintances, I am sure you can remember what it was like to see them the next day. You feel oddly close and connected to them, and what makes this even stranger is that they have no idea you even feel this way. You want to tell them, but you know they will never get it. It's as though they suddenly became one of your dearest friends but they have no memory of it— awkward.

Just watching a heroic film can make us feel empowered, which is silly, really. But that is the magic of how the human mind works. If movies only made us feel good when we were in a good mood then we would never get around to watching them, proving our circumstances don't have to change for us to feel wonderful.

You will learn to use this tool throughout your day to create wonderful feeling states exactly the way a movie can make you feel warm, hopeful, and encouraged. You already unconsciously alter your mood in various other ways all day long. Sometimes it's for the better—you turn up your favorite song, smell your favorite candle, daydream about your summer vacation, or have a dream that leaves you feeling like you visited Nirvana. At other times, you make yourself feel terrible by watching the news, listening to some political argument, or asking your tactless partner, "Does my butt look fat in these?" Either way, whether you know it or not, you have altered your brain's chemistry and, therefore, your mood. This inborn skill is what you will learn to use to your advantage—no longer blindly allowing your brain to throw your mood into a tailspin. You will learn how to plug into this powerhouse consistently on a conscious level, naturally and permanently altering your mood toward a positive sense of well-being.

The Power of Your Brain to Change Your Mind

The reason you will be able to permanently rewire your brain to focus on good things, rather than potential problems is due to something called neuroplasticity. In 1996, neuroplasticity was finally proven. This monumental breakthrough meant that the long standing belief that the human brain did not change after adolescence was all wrong. Neuroplasticity meant that the brain is not static and can change daily and even moment to moment according to what we are doing or learning. Brain areas can switch jobs, grow new cells, and even enlarge, depending on how much we use them. This discovery is the foundation of all hope regarding the brain's ability to repair damaged areas and improve itself.

Prior to this, we were taught in high school that if we drank alcohol, we would destroy brain cells that would never grow back. (Thank God that was wrong because it failed as a deterrent to our partying.) Now neuroscientists understand that every time we learn something new or even practice a skill repeatedly, the brain changes accordingly. Someone who has played piano or a stringed instrument will have a larger volume of area in brain dedicated to finger movement than the average person will have. This is neuroplasticity. On a grander scale, this process occurs in the brain of a blind person whose hearing develops way beyond what the normal range would be. The part of the brain that used to receive input from the eyes (called the occipital lobe) looks for another way to receive information, so it joins forces with the part of the brain used for hearing, increasing the amount of brainpower dedicated for hearing. Stroke victims can 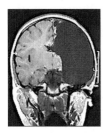 sometimes recover speech or movement because the undamaged portion of their brain begins learning the required action. However, the most magnificent illustration is that neurosurgeons have performed hundreds of hemispherectomies (removing half of a person's brain) because of disorders that are uncontrollable in any other way. Unbelievably, the surgery has no apparent effect on personality or memory. Some of the patients are now in college doing very nicely; one such person became a champion bowler, and one is a chess champion of his state. I know what you are wondering now—and the answer is no, we can't just have the sad part of the brain cut out. Thankfully, however, we won't have to.

Neuroplasticity is the light at the end of the tunnel in your search for happiness and wellbeing. It is how you will redirect your brain's focus to the hundreds of really good things that happen every day and away from its normal diet of doom and gloom. The change in focus will completely alter your emotional landscape to one of peace, contentment, and security. As you learn to see and think differently, your brain will rewire itself, causing your perception and various beliefs to change as well. Wise men and women have been telling us to do this for thousands of years. Remember the cliché "Stop and smell the roses" and the Bible verse, Philippians 4:8 that says to meditate on whatever is good, lovely, and pure? Well, science has finally caught up and proves that doing so will change our lives.

Getting Hijacked By Your Amygdala

The questions may be the most valuable part of the book, enabling you to really learn about yourself. Try not to blow past them. I know you are busy, but this is too important. The degree to which you learn about yourself will be the degree to which you have success with this program. Guaranteed!

How many times per week do you find yourself getting angry over things that you later realize were trivial?

_____

In what area does this happen most often—family, work, friends?
Can you pinpoint what situations trigger you? E.g. money, status, relationships.

_____

_____

Given what you have learned thus far, would you agree that while you are upset, chemicals are in play—chemicals that you can't control by trying to think different thoughts at that precise moment?

_____

Have you noticed that time has a way of allowing you to eventually see things differently, once you are calm?

_____

Why does this happen; can you now explain what changed?

_____

_____

Describe a time when you tried to calm down in the middle of a rage, the emotions that seemed to control you, and the thoughts that fueled it.

_____

_____

_____

_____

_____

Do you remember noticing reasonable thoughts during your explosion that you rejected because you simply didn't want to stop ranting?

_____

_____

_____

Do you find it exhausting or empowering to rant about every little thing? Have you ever tried to reset your emotional thermostat by altering your perspective?

_____

_____

Sleeping puts your thinking mind on hold. Have you found that a nap can change your mood or even the way you see a situation? If so, describe a situation when that happened.

_____

_____

Incessant Thinking

To see how random and redundant your thoughts are, please set a timer for two minutes. If you have a cell phone that has voice recording, turn it on. Take three deep, long, slow breaths (count to six for the inhale and to eight for the exhale). I want you to just listen to your breathing, but be aware of every thought that enters your mind. Say each thought aloud, record it on your phone, and then let the thought go. After two minutes are up, listen to what you recorded and write down how many thoughts are related to future events and how many thoughts relate to the past. Your goal is to notice the underlying emotions attached to these thoughts. This is not a clear process; you may see images such as old memories come to life in your mind but then miss the underlying emotion attached to them. i.e. shame, pride, anger, which can influence your mood. You may recall a conversation from that day but miss the accompanying thought of wishing you said something differently or worrying whether the other person took what you said the wrong way. Try to catch all the underlying thoughts/emotions attached to any images that pop up. See how many times you are onto the third or fourth thought before you even realize it. Guaranteed, you will need more paper for this.

_____

_____

_____

_____

_____

_____

_____

_____

_____

There is a vast difference between doing things to avoid negative feelings (which is what most of us do) and doing things to actually change those feelings into positive ones. You are going to learn to do the latter.

What kinds of behaviors do you engage in to
avoid feelings of discomfort? Write how often.

• Drinking	• Sex
• Sleeping	• Drugs/Meds
• Other	• Eating

Do you feel better or worse after doing these behaviors? Explain:

_____

_____

_____

List the things you do, if ever, to increase feelings of happiness when you are feeling negative. Also, include any new ideas that come to you (e.g., reading a book, going out with friends, communing with nature, taking a nap, calling a friend, going to the gym, listening to music, or watching a movie).

_____

Trying to just ease discomfort is not very helpful for actually improving a bad mood. However, people continue to engage in activity that holds little promise except to help you forget.

If you completed these exercises, well done! You are that much closer to feeling happy!

A•MYG•DA•LA (Latin for almond: is also referred to as lizard brain)

- Evaluates your inner and outer environment much faster than your conscious awareness can.

- Does not require your awareness.

- Retains your earliest experiences and weaves them into your ongoing experiences.

- Tends to generalize your circumstances from past specific instances.

Definitions:

Amygdala— Latin for almond. Has a primary role in the processing of emotional reactions: the amygdalae are considered part of the limbic system (the area that handles our emotions).

Neuroplasticity— The brain's ability to change. The brain can reorganize itself by forming new neural connections throughout life.

Reptilian brain— Refers to the oldest part of the human brain.

Cortisol— A hormone made in the adrenal glands.
Stress increases its production.

CHAPTER

OUR BRAIN'S PHARMACY: THE BEST PHARMACY ON EARTH

AS I HAVE EXPLAINED, WE HAVE THIS OLD PROGRAM BUILT INTO THE OLDEST PART OF THE HUMAN BRAIN. It triggers the amygdala and sends constant distress signals (SOS) at the slightest provocation to rob us of our peace and happiness. When that happens, we overreact and stress out. In this chapter, I want to delve deeper into the chemical underpinnings controlling your mood and behaviors so

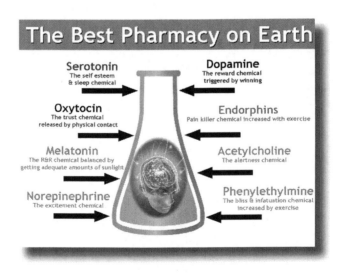

you can learn how to cut negative chemical signals off at the pass, restoring you to a sense of well-being.

Now these three names might be new; however, if you can understand the difference between octane levels at the gas pump, you can understand these as well. I am sure you will have to come back to the terms a few times to memorize them, but it will be well worth your effort.

Consider these brain chemicals like a light switch in a room. Different rooms control different moods. (I know you have a lot more than three moods; I am referring to three categories of mood.) When you feel a certain way, you will be able walk down the hall and see which light went out (brain chemical) in what room—and then you will know what to do to get it turned back on.

The first time you heard the term endorphins was likely back in the '80s. Endorphins are a brain neurotransmitter (just a big word for the way your brain sends and receives messages). This particular brain chemical is responsible for the natural high that runners can experience. But it is also associated with drugs such as heroin or morphine. Everyone was abuzz back then about how it was the reason cigarettes were so hard to quit. "Cigarettes are like morphine to your brain," people were saying.

There are many of these chemical messengers but today you are going to learn about the three that drive almost every decision you make! They are the "WHY" behind all of your behaviors, the drive behind what you call instincts and base desires.

What Fires Together, Wires Together

When your brain learns that donuts can put a smile on your face or a banana split can make you feel almost euphoric, it builds networks to reinforce these behaviors so that you never forget them.

Therefore, when you walk into a bakery and smell pastries or walk past the ice cream in your supermarket, your brain triggers certain brain chemicals, leading you to conclude that eating these things will be good for your survival. Your brain has been building neural networks dedicated to the eating of various tasty things since you were young. Every birthday, people celebrated you, complimented you, admired you, and showered you with gifts. For the finale, they gave you a giant cake with flames on it, and if that wasn't enough, they sang to you! You then consummated the moment by shoveling a giant piece of delicious, sugary carbohydrates into your mouth, so you linked the whole event together in your brain on multiple levels: food, love, fun, gifts, taste, and song!

Then we wonder why we charge the nearest bakery or ice cream shop when we are feeling down? I'm surprised we don't demand that they supply balloons and sing to us as well!

Many of your brain's connections evolved through the experiences you had personally and formed over time by watching those around you. If your dad was a big Yankees fan and you grew up seeing him get happy and excited as he watched the team play, you might find that you are now a Yankees fan having the same experience.

The brain chemicals you will learn about can lead you toward or away from experiences, people, and even food. Knowing what each one does is what will give you the upper hand when you are trying to curtail a mood. This is the crucial information that has been missing from many of the self-help books out there. Often reviewing the psychological reasons for your behavior before addressing the chemical drives that initiated them. Understanding this can save you a lot of time when trying to break habits. It is important to understand how fast these chemicals jump into action. For example, you see a commercial on TV advertising some kind of food. Before you can describe who is in the commercial, your brain has checked in to see if you are hungry. Depending on that answer, a brain chemical (dopamine) will trigger you to either move toward your refrigerator or it does nothing allowing you to stay under the blanket and wait for your show to come back on.

How We Chase "Feeling Good"

Dopamine = Drive

This is your "high" octane. It is the chemical that causes you to chase a thrill and feel excitement. It is there to tell you, *"Yeah, yeah, do that; you're gonna love this!"* Dopamine is released when an anticipated reward is due, causing you to chase what your brain thinks is good for your survival. It is the feeling you get from cocaine or from riding a roller coaster. If you are feeling listless or bored, you might try to chase some dopamine. That can result in getting into debates or arguments or venting on social media. Maybe challenging a driver on the road who annoys you, or engage in risky behaviors, like going to a bar and taking someone home you don't know well. You might do something stupid with your money, such as buy an expensive luxury item you don't really need or can't afford or throw it into a fast trade in the market. So you must be aware of these kinds of tendencies and recognize what you are craving when you feel impulsive. Behind every comfort food craving is dopamine pushing you toward that sugar, salt, or chocolate. It's the "why you can't have just one _____" (fill in your own answer).

The profile of a person driven by dopamine varies because our life experiences mold these urges and drives, See if you can relate to any of these behaviors: A person might seek out challenges or a quest. They are willing to push themselves to achieve goals because their brains give them a hit of dopamine from just the thought of reaching one.

Dopamine will push you to pursue things that are harmful and can hurt your survival if you do them long enough, such as gambling, drinking, drugs, multiple sexual partners, and many other types of behavior. Add endorphins to the mix, and you have the high that bulimics and self-mutilators experience. A much more inclusive list is in the back of this book.

Serotonin = Status

Serotonin is our "well-being" drug. It is present when we look at a sunset and feel total contentment. Serotonin evolved to tell us that our needs have been met, that we are safe and secure.

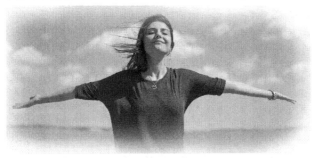

It is released when we eat a good meal, are highly praised, or accomplish a task. Serotonin gets released anytime we are considered better than others. Apparently, science has determined that there is a need for status among most species, not just humans, so thousands of years ago that status craving took the shape of producing lots of offspring,+ a drive that still dominates some cultures.

When lacking serotonin, you may feel obsolete, unimportant, empty, and (in severe cases) depressed. If you find that you are worrying about possible future events or that you are feeling vulnerable, you need serotonin. You might find yourself feeling more nervous when traveling, concerned about your safety or the safety of your loved ones. If you have ever been out socially and then suddenly wish you were at home snug in bed, you might be looking for some serotonin. Whenever you feel insecurity creeping in, you need to increase serotonin, but unless you understand that is what you need, you can do really stupid things, oblivious to why you did them. You might start pushing too hard to get ahead of others at work. You might engage in behavior such as bragging about yourself, your exploits, your material possessions, or your children. You might challenge the opinions of others or begin ranting about the plight of mankind or gorge on comfort foods that you know you should not be eating.

Oxytocin = Being loved.

Oxytocin is known as the "cuddle hormone". This neurochemical is responsible for bonding a mother with her newborn after giving birth. It is also released after sex and during cuddling, nursing, or a nurturing moment with a loved one. When people hold hands with someone or feel included in a group, oxytocin rewards them so they continue to stay close to others. People often let others win or be in charge just to keep the peace and feel more oxytocin. It motivates some to be caregivers and others to take in a stray animal. Oxytocin is released even during a simple twenty-second hug.

Therapy Dogs have become popular in hospitals and nursing homes because any patient engaging with the dog will have a spike in oxytocin, not only helping the person feel better both physically and emotionally but actually aiding in the healing process. When someone is in pain, even holding the person's hand will reduce the sensation of pain, and a recent study revealed that holding the photo of a loved one reduced even more pain than holding the person's actual hand! The lists in the back of this book will give you positive ways to trigger each neurochemical.

Dopamine= Drive, Excitement, Reward, Fun, Winning

In present-day America, the ways we experience dopamine looks very different than it did ten thousand years ago. These days it is the thrill we get on Christmas morning or on our birthdays when we are about to be showered with gifts. It is the juice that can have some people screaming at a TV, at people they don't know who are running with a ball. It is the high associated with cocaine that is so powerful it can cause a person to chase hits of the drug until their heart stops. It is the drive that pushes us to find our mate and to risk our lives if need be to hold onto that love. It is the spark we get when we are falling in love. Dopamine is released when we speed, go on a shopping spree, play sports, or do anything risky that could result in a win. It's the excitement when our team wins, at the thought of a promotion, at finding money, or while gambling or doing illegal activity. Dopamine also gets released in an infant's brain at the sound of the mother's voice. We set the stage for dopamine patterns to get hardwired into our brain throughout our lives.

For instance, if you go to an amusement park, you feel the same thrill and excitement well up inside you as an adult as you did when you were a child, even though you have no intention of riding any of the roller coasters.

Each year, many people seem to expect the same magic at the holidays as they had as children, only to be disappointed. However, despite the disappointment year after year, they seem to hold onto this expectation because of the many years the brain hardwired that holiday magic into their memory, attaching big doses of dopamine to it. So as the holiday approaches, old memories surface, releasing dopamine, telling them a reward is approaching. Being aware of why this anticipation starts can keep people from serious disappointment.

Some people pursue a career simply because of the thrilling dopamine release it brings: race car drivers, cops, and firefighters. There is a lot of dopamine released in anticipation of winning, arresting criminals, or putting out fires. Dopamine-seeking people may also be referred to as adrenaline junkies.

Dopamine is just the beginning of a complicated chain reaction meant to move you toward something. Then other neurotransmitters, such as serotonin, oxytocin, and endorphins, jump in after the experience is over to inform you, *"This was good for your survival."*

Here is an example. You go to dinner, and as you enter the restaurant, you smell delicious food; dopamine surges tell you to go toward the smell. After you eat the meal, serotonin kicks in, making you feel calm and relaxed, telling you, "Good job. You will live another day!"

Serotonin = Contentment, Safety, Confidence, Status

When you own things that you know others wish they had, serotonin is there to reward you. Today we get our serotonin fix by chasing admiration, wealth, and fame. You could say that Hollywood is the epitome of a serotonin junkie. Being adored by others makes us feel better than others, which in turn makes us feel safe and secure. On the annoying side, it can make us know-it-alls, cause us to brag or relentlessly post pictures on Facebook of each day of our vacation.

Serotonin can have an adverse effect on your relationships,

much more than dopamine or oxytocin can. When you notice serotonin taking a dip, you may do any of the following: make a joke at someone else's expense, insinuate that you make more money than someone else, or resist giving in during an argument because it is too uncomfortable to let anyone think you don't know what you are talking about. You might also mention the important person you had lunch with, announce your children's latest successes, or start using a tanning booth by December. Once you know why you are doing these things, you can be more aware when the need for serotonin creeps in so you can resist the urge to hijack the conversation or boast because you need to feel better than others in the room. Although serotonin junkies are egomaniacs, on the flip side, serotonin can bring out the best in you making you the first one to say "yes" when asked to volunteer or help someone. Serotonin is the reason for feeling a deep need to rescue others and placing a high premium on the plight of humanity. A depletion of serotonin will cause depression and is thought to be responsible for anxiety disorders. This is why most antidepressants are used to increase or maintain serotonin levels.

Being singled out by a superior will put you on a serotonin cloud, but it also explains why you might not feel very good when it happens to a coworker because that can trigger fears of being rejected, left out, or ignored all of which is a direct result of your serotonin dropping.

Oxytocin = Being Loved, Sex, Bonding

When you are lacking in oxytocin, it is common to feel lonely and isolated to varying degrees. This can cause you to sleep with someone you don't know well or reconnect with an ex-lover you know is unhealthy for you. You may rescue an animal that you really are not ready to take on as a pet. It can also propel you to become involved with groups simply because they make you feel connected.

Many don't know that laughter is not only fun but also one of the oldest traits humans have. Every culture in the world partakes in laughter. For laughter to survive this long means that evolution determined it was essential to our survival. Why it is as important as our other basic needs such as companionship and food, has been something scientists have been trying to understand. A good hard laugh releases oxytocin and endorphins, making you feel connected to those you are laughing with. This is why one of the first ways we try to engage with children or babies is to get them to smile and laugh with us. There is an immediate connection when they do. If you have ever been in a comedy club, you will notice that as people

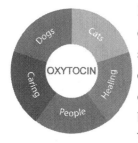

laugh, they often look around the room for connection with the others laughing. You will also notice that you laugh less when watching comedy by yourself than when you are with others. Your brain's goal is not the laughing but the bonding and connecting with others. You might recall wanting to watch a funny movie with someone who you thought would appreciate the humor, even though you had already seen the movie several times. That is because the connection you experience with that person is much more appealing than the movie itself. Children connect through humor by making adults laugh. They tell us jokes, act silly, or (as they get older and as my nephew liked to do) recount the comedy they have seen in movies verbatim.

When I was in my forties and unmarried, my friendships took on a greater role in my life; my friends were like my family. Having any kind of riff with any of them left me miserable, as my brain would send vague messages that my life and survival were being threatened.

It should be noted that the sexes can differ a bit in how they relate to these neurochemicals. For instance, it's fair to say that little girls are generally wired to maintain friendships, and they can feel devastated when their friendship is rejected. Girls are wired more for socialization—and communication. We girls love connecting, and because oxytocin is a part of that, we are much more prone to seek the comfort of others and enjoy social gatherings. It is thought that because we give birth we have more oxytocin. Oxytocin allows us to read the emotions of others so we can connect with them better. Autistic people have a deficit in oxytocin, making it very hard for them to interpret the faces and emotions of others.

Boys have more testosterone and can be more driven by dopamine, constantly steering them toward assertive encounters in which they try to find their security by dominating others. They are less interested in connection and more focused on their independence.

Remember this when men and women work together. Most of the time they are wired to have very different goals. Woman derive their sense of success by how interconnected they are, while men derive their sense of success by how independent they are.

This is why some women can get taken advantage of by ruthless salesmen. I usually bring the most frugal guy I know with me when buying big items that require negotiating like a car, and I am hardly a wimp. Without realizing it, a woman can find herself wanting to please the salesman, not wanting to let him down, so to speak. We are not weak; we are just supercharged to connect with those around us. Again, I am generalizing, so don't shoot me if you are not in that category.

In Summary

It is harder than you think to simply ignore these instinctual drives. Becoming aware of them, though, is the first step to learning to alter your subconscious behavior. These neurochemicals are not released exclusively of one another, and their effects can vary, depending on the part of your brain or body they are released in. That is why feeling attracted to a new potential mate due to the dopamine release does not feel quite the same as the dopamine release you get when your team wins.

Fifty percent of all dopamine and 5 percent of serotonin are made in your brain. Your gut produces the other 50 percent of the dopamine and 95 percent of your serotonin! That is why following your gut feeling can really pay off. Many scientists refer to it as "the other brain."

The crux of this book is to understand why and how these chemicals rise and fall. You can learn to trigger these mood-altering chemicals in your brain when you want to do so, which is how you will learn to be happy.

As your attitudes, values and priorities change throughout your life, these brain chemicals follow suit. This is why you are able to change behaviors and even longstanding habits—because the underpinning of every behavior is a brain chemical (or neurochemical) rewarding you or punishing you for your choices.

Let's look at a few simple examples of how changing what you believe can change your brain. When I started going to the gym, I was frustrated and annoyed that I had to give up my time to do it. Just the mere thought of going to the gym reduced my dopamine and serotonin levels and released cortisol. However, after a year of going to the gym, I had retrained my mind to accept the sacrifice of time to get back in shape. As my body began to make small improvements, I felt better about how I looked, which released serotonin. Soon I found that the mere thought of going to the gym now released dopamine, moving me toward the activity of working out. Remember: **dopamine=drive and motivation.**

Dieting is another example of how beliefs/perception can alter people's experience and outcome. In the first few months, many individuals become frustrated that they can't eat the way others do. They may believe they are being deprived or even punished, causing a lowering of the feel-good chemicals, dopamine, and serotonin. However, if they stick with it, and begin to lose the weight, they feel better about themselves. Then their brains release hits of dopamine and serotonin whenever they just think about their new eating habits. (Why people go off their diet is a subject for an entire book). The job of these neurochemicals is to make us feel good when we do things that benefit us. The issue is that sometimes we have to teach our brains WHAT IS GOOD for us!

Anti-Stress Vaccine

When we were kids, we played tag, a game that meant running around trying not to let another kid tag you. When you felt someone was getting close, you ran as fast as you could to home base, a specific spot in the yard such as the front steps, and you would yell, "Safe!" Well, there is a SAFE place for us too, a condition in the brain that will keep us safe from most stress. It is a mind-set in which the brain finds it impossible to get angry. You may say, "Really? Is there such a thing?" Yes there is. What life event or emotion makes it nearly impossible to become angry, or frustrated? When your rich uncle leaves you a million dollars? After sex? The real answer is being filled with gratitude and appreciation. I am not being philosophical. There is a scientific, chemical basis for this. When you are filled with overwhelming appreciation and gratitude, your brain is flooded with all three very powerful neurotransmitters: dopamine, oxytocin, and serotonin. I refer to them as DOS. Now there are about eight main feel-good chemicals, as you can see in the diagram on the first page of this chapter, but in this book, DOS will be the focus because when your brain is flooded with these three chemicals, it is immunized from stress. Getting annoyed would be like trying to start a fire with wet logs.

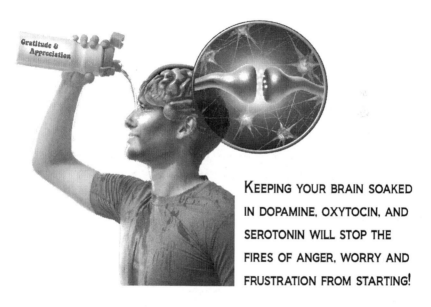

KEEPING YOUR BRAIN SOAKED IN DOPAMINE, OXYTOCIN, AND SEROTONIN WILL STOP THE FIRES OF ANGER, WORRY AND FRUSTRATION FROM STARTING!

How Do You Relieve The Pain?

We human beings are just like addicts, making decisions from one moment to the next based on 2 questions: What will give me the greatest amount of pleasure right now or the least amount of discomfort? Every situation—physical, emotional, or social—is fueled, directed, and regulated by the drug effect we are seeking from the brain's own chemical pharmacy, and this pharmacy is open twenty-four hours a day! The timely release of the "feel good" chemicals in the brain underpins a healthy emotional balance.

However, scientist know that we humans often take bigger steps to **avoid** the pain of feeling bad than to **pursue** feeling good and you are going to learn to reverse that. When we are trying to ease discomfort we may chase a hit of any of these three neurochemicals, by reaching for ice cream, having sex, or sitting down to watch a good movie; the multi-taskers in the group may attempt all three at the same time. However, as we all have experienced the feelings are short-lived. That is because these neurochemicals have a job, and that is to push our behavior in a direction, not put us in a "good mood". That good feeling is just like the proverbial carrot, always tempting us to chase another short-lived buzz and it can become a vicious cycle. We don't want the buzz we want a sense of wellbeing.

Feeling good, happy, safe, secure, and loved, tell our brain that we have a better chance of survival. The negative effects of cortisol and adrenaline tell us that we are in danger of NOT surviving. Without realizing it we repeatedly activate all of these chemicals more often with our thoughts and beliefs than by out right behavior. By making subconscious decisions literally second by second, we are triggering them. Let's refer to our subconscious as the "back room".

Although it feels like we live under one steady stream of stress it doesn't work that way. Just like the good chemicals of DOS have to be triggered repeatedly, we are repeatedly triggering our stress response. As each moment arises with its own unique conditions our subconscious sends out the orders to: trust, like, love, or distrust, don't like, and fear. But with our brains favoring the negative, we more often fall on the dark side of disliking and fear. We now have to make *conscious* decisions, these will come from the "head office". When you learn to make conscious decisions all day long that support positive perspectives you will be replacing the constant stream of negative perspectives that are plaguing you all day long. This alters your mood toward a good one, relieving you of the urge to ease discomfort with bad choices. This is why you *can no longer trust your autopilot decision-making processes coming from the "back office"*.

Just as we are all different from one other, so are our cravings. The same situation can make two people react very differently. For example, playing the slots at a casino will give some people a hit of dopamine in anticipation of a win. For others it triggers cortisol/anxiety because they anticipate a loss.

Two siblings are dreading a big report soon due at school. At the mere thought of starting it, both feel anxious. But one will avoid it and procrastinate, putting off the anxiety. The other child, although anxious, knows that completing the project will alleviate her anxiety, and the thought of that triggers dopamine, so that child starts the project right away. If you are a parent it can help seeing much of your children's behavior from this standpoint as it will aid you greatly in understanding them not to mention helping them to understand themselves.

Here is a typical *subconscious process*; One starts their day off with a to-do list because they know that as they cross things off this list, they will get bursts of serotonin. One problem, it was all outdoor work and it has begun to drizzle. Without a back up plan the threat of no productivity reduces their serotonin, and in a blink, dopamine is driving them toward a fatty or sugary treat. Frustration is now felt stopping the flow of new creative tasks that can be tackled. Annoyed they plop down in front of the TV and wait for the rain to stop. By time it has, other chemicals have come on line triggering guilt, for sitting around, anger at the weather, and a sense the day will be lost. Now all of this negative emotion has to be overcome. Two choices; get off the couch and get busy, which will trigger everything they need to feel better or they will grab whatever will *ease* the discomfort the *fastest* which may be a beer, a shopping spree or a nap. Being ignorant of why their mood is fluctuating can cause them to lose the whole day and have no idea why.

Avoid engaging in unconscious, negative behaviors that can sabotage your day. The sudden desire for a cookie will seem innocent enough, but then you devour the whole bag. (OK, I devour the whole bag.) Often your body hides it's craving for serotonin in the form of some kind of treat. But once you know this you can make better choices to find your *happy place.*

Shopping sprees are one of the more popular ways to chase dopamine and serotonin. See if any part of this story sounds familiar. You decide you need a new TV. You enter the store, and your brain begins to feel almost giddy as you are struck by the colors on the large screens and the lifelike sounds that seem to surround your body. Suddenly your brain is filling with dopamine. Within seconds, you are envisioning having this powerful experience in the comfort of your own home; images of having friends over to wow them on game day fill your head. Your dopamine level is soaring as it screams, "Go! Go! Go!" Before you know it, you are divulging your annual salary to a complete stranger so you can purchase the entire home theater system on credit. You close the deal by telling yourself that your payment will be so small that your budget will hardly notice. *Well done!* However, brace yourself because if you begin to feel guilty and worried about this ridiculous overindulgence, your serotonin will drop like a rock and you will feel awful. That's called buyer's remorse; it stings and turns that delicious high-flying sensation into a sickening feeling in the pit of your stomach. Your body is replacing that nice serotonin and dopamine with cortisol. Yuck! You go from loving life to having your brain tell you that your life is in danger! The cure? Return the item? No, that will also decrease serotonin, so that is out. What most do is buy something else to keep the high alive and offset the cortisol. Add some Blu-ray movies, and you might feel a bit better. Well done, junkie!

Just like an addict we can be unaware of how we are hurting ourselves and others with our impulsivity. Then, fed up with the guilt and the judgment from our friends and family (cortisol), we opt for new resolves, confess to a spiritual adviser, or buy a new self-help book.

If you can relate to any of this you may have been told you were undisciplined, self-centered, or immature. Ideally, people should grow out of this impulsivity, and most do, but not always in every area. Some of us still cling to behaviors such as shopping, cheating, temper tantrums, or taking risks with our life or money. Only when we finally understand what has been driving our behavior will we find ways to remedy it. *(It is imperative that you understand all the negative ways you have been trying to release these neurochemicals, so I have detailed lists in the back of this book.)*

As people age, their neurochemical favorite can change. People in their forties often laugh about how they used to like going out on the weekends because now their favorite thing to do is work in their garden or curl up with a good book. Young people can't comprehend this as being fun or enjoyable because their taste for dopamine still exceeds their taste for serotonin. What has happened is that the brain's appetite for dopamine-type pleasures has traded itself in for serotonin-type pleasures. Rather than excitement and thrill, these people would rather feel secure and stable enjoying the pleasure of their own home, a choice that people in their teens and twenties don't typically have.

My goal is to teach you how to experience all the wonderful feelings of well-being by absorbing healthy and uplifting experiences in a way that you've never done before. Like I said our brain comes pre-wired to overlook most positive experiences unless those experiences are immense. The change will not take long or require much effort. You are going to learn how to pause for 10 to 15 seconds to create the feelings you really want, and this will change your life forever. You will start feeling happier and calmer and will walk with a sense of well-being every day if you are willing to commit to this process of awareness in ten to fifteen-second increments. How much faster could "instant" be?

Learning how to obtain a more consistent release of these chemicals in healthy ways is all you need to do to be happier. The process entails simply becoming aware of all the goodness around you and allowing your brain to create new neural networks that reinforce their goodness for you, just like it did about birthday cakes or your favorite sports team years ago.

Now at first, your limbic system may not view these good things as requirements for survival, which is why you will have to allow ten seconds for your thinking brain to focus on their goodness, giving your limbic system time to respond with one or all three neurochemicals that you will experience as emotions. However, once you do this a few times, your brain will note your focus and switch on your reticular activating system, which means it knows to look for more of these positive experiences! After only three weeks, your brain will begin to see more good events in your life than negative ones! (But I don't want to get ahead of myself; there is more for you to understand.)

With a few scientifically proven techniques and practices, you will instantly start having new emotional experiences that will release dopamine, oxytocin, and serotonin (DOS). Your brain's primary focus will no longer be the fear of a lion in the bushes or the bill in the mail. Your goal is to build up a reserve of these good feelings and fill your synapses with DOS. Once you are making a consistent effort to feel these good experiences throughout your day, your over reactive amygdala will begin to quiet down, allowing you to let many problems roll off your back. You will then experience an increase in your overall feelings of happiness and well-being. *Remember to keep your brain soaked in these good chemicals so the panic fires can't start.*

How Do You Engage With DOS?

The time you invest in thinking through the following questions will give you a deeper understanding of the roles these chemicals have been playing and how they have been affecting your behavior.

Describe 3 positive events from the past that you have experienced **dopamine**.

1)
2)
3)

Describe 3 negative events from the past that you have chased **dopamine**.

1)
2)
3)

Describe 3 positive behaviors/patterns that you use to get your **dopamine** fix.

1)
2)
3)

Describe 3 negative behaviors/patterns that you use to get your **dopamine** fix.

1)

2) _____

3) _____

Describe 3 positive events from the past that you have experienced **oxytocin.**

1) _____

2) _____

3) _____

Describe 3 negative events from the past that you have used to get **oxytocin fix.**

1) _____

2) _____

3) _____

Describe 3 positive behaviors/patterns that you use to get your **oxytocin** fix.

1) _____

2) _____

3) _____

Describe 3 negative behaviors/patterns that you use to get your **oxytocin** fix.

1) _____

2) _____

3) _____

Describe 3 positive events from the past you have experienced **serotonin.**

1) _____

2) _____

3) _____

Describe 3 negative events from the past where you experienced **serotonin.**

1) _____

2) _____

3) _____

Describe 3 positive behaviors/patterns that you use to get your **serotonin** fix.

1) _____

2) _____

3) _____

Describe 3 negative behaviors that you use to get your **serotonin** fix.

1) _____

2) _____

3) _____

From the exercises above, can you determine which neurochemical you might favor? This is not black and white, by any means, and you may be biased toward different chemicals at different times of the month or season. But these exercises will help you get a handle on where your hot buttons are. It might be easier to find your favorite neurochemical by asking yourself what events upset you more. *Whatever upsets you more is probably a chemical you favor most.*

Dopamine: Losing in any type of game like video, cards, chess, or a sport you play, having your favorite team lose, being bored, feeling the need for excitement, craving risks like racing, skydiving, gambling.

Oxytocin: Having your best friend think you let him or her down. Having an argument with someone you love, being without your pet, being lonely, being left out or rejected.

Serotonin: Having your boss unhappy with you, seeing someone else get praise or a promotion at work, not being able to go on vacation, feeling jealous of material possessions, feeling unsafe or threatened, feeling dumb or embarrassed.

Try to organize them in order of importance at the various ages of your life. See if you can pinpoint the years in which your behavior revealed different cravings for dopamine, oxytocin, or serotonin. Example: climbing the corporate ladder in your thirties but putting family first in your forties..

5-20 Years Old

1 _____

2 _____

3 _____

20-40 Years Old _____

1 _____

2 _____

3 _____

40- Older _____

1 _____

2 _____

3 _____

You may discover that with maturity, your concept of pleasure probably has changed. For instance, the thrill of going to an amusement park (dopamine) may be replaced by a desire to be on the beach with a good book (serotonin). Also, with age comes the desire to be with one chosen partner instead of hanging out with several friends in order to get your oxytocin and serotonin.

CHAPTER

How Our Culture Stands In The Way of Our Happiness

To begin gaining control over our negative bias and redirect it toward the positive, we must understand that we humans like to make sense of our behavior. And sometimes at any cost. So for thousands of years, we have dreamed up some good reasons behind our overwhelming obsession to worry and stress out. These so-called good reasons can stand in our way until we see them for the illusions they are. When planting, we have to prepare the ground by first removing the weeds. In that same way, there are three types of weeds or barriers that we need to remove before we begin our journey toward happiness. These barriers can hold us back from embracing happiness, and we need to understand them:

- **Human habits and beliefs**
- **Psychological obstacles**
- **Physiological barriers**

All three present themselves in both overt and covert ways that we need to identify before we can remove them.

Human Habits and Beliefs

Myth One: I would be happy if ...

Most people believe our environment and events control our moods. Our culture teaches us that we need a reason to be happy. That little uptight, responsible voice in our heads says, **"What right do you have to feel happy if your life is so hard?"** Or **"You can be happy when you —"get a promotion, lose weight, get married/or become single, or have more money."** Waiting until we have a reason to be happy is like chasing the proverbial carrot at the end of the stick or waiting for tomorrow, which never actually arrives. We are programmed to believe that by being serious, with the laser focused on our problems, we will somehow handle them better and make them disappear faster. We carry around a deep-seated belief that there is a proper time and place to be happy, and it certainly does not exist in the middle of our problems or trials or before our dreams are realized. It is as though we are an angry parent standing over ourselves, saying, *"Wipe that smirk off your face; this isn't funny!"* This is another false belief, the truth is life goes better for us if we are positive and happy, not if we are feeling like an overstressed victim. Besides, if we really believed this lie that our lives have to be good before we can feel any kind of happiness, then liquor stores would close. We always chase some sort of relief, regardless of the crap that is going on. Evolution has designed us to feel like crap when things go wrong so we will put forth whatever herculean effort is needed to save our own asses. Therefore we make the choice to hold onto our anger, rage, disappointment, and frustration. The choice may be subconscious, but it's there.

Ahh, do you want to slam the book shut yet? I used to hate when people said that to me! It sounded like recycled platitudes that I wanted to shove...well, you get the idea. Remember that much more is going on under the surface of your awareness than you currently understand yet. Have you ever seen a child who is upset or pouting? Do you remember the adults around the child trying to get him or her to laugh as the child visibly fought the urge to smile? Why do children do that rather than giving in? Because to give in and smile would negate the seriousness of their feelings; who would take them seriously ever again? Even a young child of three years old seems able to figure that one out.

Well, we are not too different from that child. When frustrated, way down deep we actually make a subconscious choice to **not allow** happiness or a lightheartedness into that moment because we are wired and brought up to believe that to do so would somehow be opposed to fixing the issue at hand. It feels almost irresponsible. Not to mention that taking our problems with a grain of salt may feel similar to encouraging these problems to resurface. Let me explain.

I remember waiting in line behind a mom and her two-year-old little boy. He had big blue eyes and seemed to be studying me. I gave him a warm smile, and he responded with an ear-to-ear grin... then he flipped me the bird! After the initial shock, I couldn't help but let out a laugh. At two years old, he meant nothing by it other than to make his mom crazy and complete strangers laugh. Now, we all know that laughing is the worst thing you can do. His mom seemed to know instinctively what he had done, and although she was furious with him, he seemed more interested in me (I was now trying to hold back the laughter). I guess he was willing to forgo some oxytocin bonding with his mom for this dose of serotonin and oxytocin he was getting from me. I had inadvertently encouraged this outrageous behavior and had to apologize to his mother for not helping her. Laughing was like putting my stamp of approval on her child's behavior. It made me wonder if that perspective haunts us a bit when we try to take life's antics lightly. I realized after I thought about it, that I feared my lack of outrage over my troubles could encourage more of them to show up. Dumb, I know, life isn't watching, going, "Oh, really, you think that is funny?" As it hurls more problems at you. In fact, it's the opposite. Letting go of your frustration will alter your energy field so that fewer problems show up.

I remember once driving home from work and being really ticked off about something at work when suddenly a song came on that I loved. I remember feeling for a fleeting moment how easy it would be to just switch gears and start singing, but I didn't dare. I was furious at some coworker, and the "audience" in my head listening to my tirade would think I was really nuts if I just started singing as though nothing were wrong. *But nothing was wrong!* Not at that very moment. I was still arguing my point from a discussion that had ended two hours earlier. Is that crazier than bursting into a song?

Your amygdala is far from forgetful, and it loves the sound of sirens in the night. Feeling the effects of cortisol each time you remember the problem convinces you that you should keep ranting; *surely the offenders will show up any minute now to admit they were wrong and you were right!*

The next stage is to support this ingrained insane behavior, by contriving elaborate reasons to justify our ranting, worrying, panic and the resulting stress.

I grew up in a house where occasionally yelling about problems was considered a viable way to solve them. Much to my mother's dismay, I personally mastered this.

Like the parent who stares at her child kicking and screaming on the floor, so does life observe us, grown children, throwing tantrums because some aspect of life did not go as we *expected*—as if that will change anything! (More on expectations later.)

To change your situation, you have to battle your ever-so-reactive amygdala constantly telling you to be armed and anxious. This behavior is similar to racing down the highway speeding only because you are afraid of cops and don't want them to see you. But the faster you drive to avoid a cop, the more likely one is to spot you speeding. That fearful behavior is what creates the stress you fear so much. *Ninety-nine percent of the time, it is the critical, self-hating judge in your head that demands your frustration and indignation and not the actual situation you are facing.*

Everyone has his or her own brew of defensive reactions, from worrying, yelling, and crying to overworking, drinking, sleeping, and complaining to anyone who will listen. I hope you realize these behaviors/tantrums are full of empty promises and examine these hardwired misguided reactions more objectively. Once you see this lie exposed—that getting upset will somehow help you—your behavior will begin to change.

Where exactly in the framework of your brain is this choice to react differently? Well your powerful subconscious always has a host of options available, but the trick is getting that info up to your thinking, conscious brain to make use of it.

Have you ever had a bad day only to go to sleep and have a really happy, amazing dream? You wake up with this feeling that something wonderful happened, and you wish you could harness that feeling and take it with you all day. Why is your brain perfectly capable of making you feel that blissful while you are sleeping? Because you couldn't argue with it; that critical judge was asleep! Now you need to learn to do this when you are awake. Here is a cornerstone truth: **your brain does not need a reason to be happy; it**

<u>**needs only your mind's permission to do so!**</u>

Every day a smile, a compliment, or a hug has the power to release waves of comforting dopamine, oxytocin and serotonin, but we say "Now is not the time!" And go on punishing ourselves, believing that somehow, being stressed out will give us an advantage in figuring out our problems. This is a lie hardwired into the brain!

The truth is something as simple as a compliment holds the most promise for making you feel great. Mark Twain knew this power; he once said, "I can live two months on a good compliment."

Myth Two: Money : Many of us believe money would solve most of our problems. We all have the dream of hitting the lottery and having our money problems disappear, assuming that will make us happier. However, a very well known study was done to find out how true that was for people. What they found was that those who won the lottery described themselves as being "less happy or as happy" six months later than they were before they won. They then researched people who were left paralyzed after an accident. Many of those people were actually as happy if not happier than they had been the day before their accident. How could that possibly be? **Because our situations do not determine our happiness.**

Your amygdala will look for problems regardless of how much money you have. Lottery winners are still obsessed over every problem, real or feared. However, the paraplegic, on the other hand, has now found **appreciation/gratitude** in the small successes of even mundane tasks that you and I take for granted, from putting on shoes to holding a fork or feeding himself. Remember, people get a serotonin hit every time they feel they have accomplished any kind of task, and in this case the paraplegics are very grateful for what they *can* do. Of course they would prefer to be able to walk, but that does not affect their mood to the extent that one might expect.

I had the opportunity to see this firsthand at a physical

therapy center for disabled children. For over ten years, I have observed 99 percent of the kids from age six to fifteen being the happiest, most joyful children I have ever seen. I mean on a scale of one to ten, these kids are a twelve! It mystified me for years; then I learned that they radiate a happiness and excitement because every day they applaud themselves for accomplishing simple tasks, allowing the love of those around them to touch them deeply. They relish each success. Their secret is what neuroscience understands today...**that brief, momentary releases of dopamine, oxytocin, and serotonin throughout the day will stifle our usual overreaction so that life's setbacks seem much less threatening.** The relief we have been seeking has been in our brain all along; we have always had the best pharmacy, and soon we will learn how to write our own scripts.

Psychological Obstacles *(Misery Loves Company)*

I have a question for you. If I could give you a pill that would render you calm with a sense of peace throughout the day, a pill with no side effects that would leave you smiling during confrontations with colleagues, family, or even your boss, would you take it? Well, most people would. So for a moment, close your eyes and imagine you are at your desk or home, and a coworker or family member comes in upset and anxious. The situation is serious but hardly life threatening. You listen intently but feel as calm as if you were sitting at the beach. How would your coworker or family member react? Would he or she say, "Wow you being calm is so refreshing, I feel so much better?" Hell no!

They will most likely get upset that you aren't flipping out like they are. But why? Because it has been ingrained in us that drama and overreaction (in essence, adrenaline and cortisol) will ensure a better outcome for everyone by creating a panicked, get-off-your asses scenario. Being calm might even be perceived as not caring, leaving you feeling disconnected. When your boss is yelling at you from across his desk and wants to see you tremble, sitting there too calmly could backfire. There is a stigma with being too chill. If people are freaking out, they expect you to jump on that emotional roller coaster and ride it with them. It validates their outburst and gives them comfort that they are not alone with the problem.

Have you ever expressed anger over a political issue or some other kind of injustice only to be met with a nonchalant, who cares attitude? That can be just as upsetting as someone disagreeing with you. Make no mistake about it, without serious effort to override this tendency, you are wired to freak out and run or freak out and fight—but either way, to freak out.

Monkey See Monkey Do

There are special neurons, which reside in various parts of our brain, called mirror neurons. They are there so we can learn to mimic others' of actions and read their emotions. How they do this is when we watch other human do things, these mirror neurons fire exactly as if we were doing the same action. This is a big part of the reason we feel that we should behave the way others do in emotional moments. For example just picturing someone hitting their thumb with a hammer will cause us to wince. It is why we yawn when someone else does or clap when others begin to do so. These powerful neurons help us empathize with others. They also seem to be behind the phenomenon of a mob yelling to a suicide jumper to "jump" or a whole crowd freezing when someone falls or gets mugged or how about the mobs of people who get so worked up into a frenzy that they trample other human beings just to start shopping for the holidays! When they try to rationalize this behavior, they have no plausible explanation other than, "they did what everyone else did".

Mirror neurons are behind our love of watching movies or TV shows and reading a juicy novel. It is why we can get lost in them as the same emotions well up in us, along with the corresponding neurochemicals: dopamine, serotonin, and even oxytocin. This is also the enjoyment behind watching sports. Our brains are firing as if we were running down the field, all the while triggering our dopamine. If there is painful contact with one of the players, everyone says, "Ohhh," as if we somehow feel it.

Have you ever put the TV on with nothing in mind to watch? You begin to flip through the channels and come across a movie you

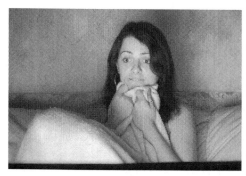

have seen five or ten times before, such as, Top Gun, Godfather, any one of the Rocky movies (add your own here), and you stop surfing and start watching. Why when you can almost lip-sync some of the scenes; there are no surprises. For one; if the characters feel a sense of triumph then so will you. Not a bad pay off for just lounging on your couch in the middle of the day! We all have a deep desire to identify, relate, and connect (IRC). That makes your brain feel safe, protected, calm, and secure, removing any sense of loneliness.

I was at a store checking out when I overheard the cashier telling a story to another customer. "I can't believe it; she gave him everything when he had nothing, and now he is cheating on her!" She was so emotionally invested that I thought for sure she knew this couple personally. Then I heard her follow up with, "I love this book; I can't get enough of it!" Really? Did she even realize that she was commenting on the behavior of people who did not exist? That she was getting emotional over actions that never took place except on the pages of a fictitious book? Of course she did, but when we humans invest our emotion and are moved by stories, real or not, it is as though they deserve our full attention. Most of us don't know what a mirror neuron is, but we are controlled by them just the same.

These mirror neurons are very active during video games as players' brains fire as if they were in the game. This is the compelling argument regarding the violence in these games. Our limbic brain does not distinguish between real or fake; only the mature prefrontal cortex can do that. That is why we can be moved to tears or feel our bodies tense up just by watching a bunch of images on a screen twenty feet away. Connecting us one to another through mirror neurons was evolution's way of increasing our chances of survival. Who could have predicted that thousands of years later, much of our entertainment would depend on the use of our mirror neurons?

This is a powerful obstacle to overcome if you are trying to stay calm while everyone around you is yelling, "The sky is falling!" You will have to fight your instincts because you will naturally want to feel what others feel. You need to realize that you can't save everyone else. This is about you taking charge of your emotional environment and staying as stress free as possible. Eventually your reaction will be appreciated and even sought out by others and there certainly is no better example for your children to see.

Physiological Barriers— Threats Trump Happiness

For the past ten thousand years, the threat of danger had more impact on our survival than good experiences; therefore, our amygdala was primed to label most experiences as dangerous and has continued to do so right up until present day. *We were built to last, not for lasting happiness, which is why we learn faster from pain than from pleasure.* Each time something happens that we don't like, cortisol magnifies the feeling, embedding it into our memory as a threat of some kind.

For example, your boss gives you a stellar review, but at the very end, he says, "The only thing I would like to see improved is_____." Yet after your meeting, all your brain focuses on is the one thing he wants you to improve.

We all tend to do this, regardless of the feedback or the source of it. The brain digs out the negative comment; sometimes it may even dig through a positive one and think, "Hmm, but what was he really trying to say?" We tell ourselves that we do this because we just want to improve but that is contrived crap! The real reason we do it is that the brain interprets any slightly negative feedback from another person as us being at risk for being "kicked out of the tribe."

Having a simple disagreement even with someone you love can switch the amygdala to the fight-or-flight position. You enter into a discussion in which you expect the person to agree with you. Then when the person doesn't, cortisol releases, causing an immediate shutting down of reasonable thinking and processing. Cortisol interrupts the prefrontal cortex as it tells your brain, **"Your life is in danger; this is no time to be thinking!"** So you raise your voice, yell, and take on aggressive body posture. Your whole body is reacting as if the other person is a threat to your life. That is a pretty crappy way to feel around your spouse or best friend. This is why arguments rarely prove fruitful and is why discussing topics such as religion and politics is so dangerous. No one wants to hear what you think unless you agree with them.

Part of cortisol's job is to help you remember disagreeable

experiences. It is there to tell you, "Hey, remember this; your life could depend on it in the future!"

I was watching a debate between two scholars. I sided with one scholar because I thought he made a much better argument. The other scholar was flippant, arrogant, and demeaning, all of which I found distasteful—yet I remembered with great detail! I remembered very few details from the scholar I liked. This amazed me. I remembered the guy I totally disagreed with, who I thought behaved like a buffoon, all because my cortisol had heightened the experience, embedding it into my memory. This is why in relationships, it is easier to recall the hurtful things said rather than all of the loving ones.

Like I mentioned earlier if you had a particularly difficult childhood, your amygdala will tend to be larger and even more primed to overreaction. Your emotions will be more dramatic and quicker to react, and your thoughts over concerns can be like a needle stuck on a scratch. You will replay an insult or argument in your mind sometimes for days, thousands of times, embedding that hurt in your brain over and over.

Thousands of years ago, when your life was suddenly in real danger you responded by running like hell, and then you forgot about it. You did not analyze it to death; you were still breathing, and that was good enough. Today all you do is analyze, anticipate, prepare for, and worry about every single thing your amygdala flags as dangerous. So when you are waiting for test results or you get that unexpected bill, the chant begins, "You must be prepared!" Simply believing there will be a positive outcome feels irresponsible.

Studies have shown that 85 percent of the time, the object of our worries and anxiety never materializes—85 percent! That is a huge amount of wasted energy! Remember, *nothing is ever as bad as it feels.*

Discovery of Beliefs and Patterns of Behavior

Name any situations in which you have been waiting for change to give yourself permission to relax and be happy.

_____

_____

_____

_____

_____

_____

_____

List how long you have been waiting for each change.

_____

_____

_____

_____

_____

Have you ever felt that you could just let anger go before it overtook you? Did you give in and let the anger go or allow the anger to build? Can you describe why you made either choice and whether you were happy with it?

_____

_____

Who in your life would not appreciate you being calm when they are upset?

_____

_____

_____

How does it make you feel when you are upset and others remain calm?

_____

_____

_____

How would you feel if you could distance yourself from the drama of others?

_____

Have you ever allowed yourself to get caught up in an emotional moment only because those around you were doing so? If so, describe the experience and what it felt like.

_____

_____

_____

Circle how often do you dissect a compliment from a superior or loved one to find any negative message or insinuation?

Once in a While	Often	All the Time	Almost Never

Describe a time when you were told you were doing a great job, **but**... and then could only focus on what ever issue followed that "but".

_____

_____

_____

How often do you find your needle stuck, obsessing over a comment or conversation in your head? Circle:

Can't Remember	3x A week	3x A month	Almost Never	Everyday

List who you most often get your needle stuck with?

_____

_____

Where do you most often do this (e.g., car, bathroom, bed)? Keep in mind that wherever you do it most is where you are the least present.

_____

_____

Describe the types of situations that you try not to worry about, e.g. health, money, relationships but your mind continues going back to it repeatedly, speculating outcomes? Describe and note whether the problems were ever as bad as you feared.

_____

_____

_____

_____

_____

What three types of situations are the hardest for you to let go?

1._____

_____

2._____

_____

3._____

_____

When has speculation about outcomes ever come to fruition or excessive worry ever proven to fix one of your problems?

_____

_____

Women Are More Emotionally Perceptive

The connectivity between the left and right amygdala is 18 percent larger in women than in men, with numerous studies indicating that women are far more emotionally and socially perceptive than men are. This is why women are quick to interpret the actions and emotions of others. It is also why, at the end of a party, a wife's question to her husband about whether he noticed or could he tell_____ is met with a blank look or a retort such as "Why do you care?"

4

Problems Are In The Eye of The Beholder

Understand this fact: it is your perspective that will determine if something is good or bad. *"It's never the problem; the issue is how you SEE the problem"*. Your happiness will be a result of choices you make to see the world in a certain way. And we make those choices within every second. This is why so many studies repeatedly prove that 90 percent of our problems stem from how we see things. The philosophical question "Is the glass half full or half empty?" Does not do justice to the power of perspective. The simple truth is that events happen—what makes them bad or good is simply what you decide to *think* or *believe* about them. I am struck by how people see an approaching blizzard so differently. Some (like me) who have no use for snow, don't want to look at it or drive in it and will usually put on an ocean soundtrack. Meanwhile, others will be excited because it means great conditions for skiing; they will take pictures and post about how beautiful it is. (I tend to think they have too much time on their hands.) The snow says two entirely different things to each of us according to what we like and want.

Beauty may be in the eye of the beholder, but so are problems. That can be hard to swallow; we want our anger and frustration validated, not debunked as a figment of our perception! Most of us have been building stories for years around why things happened. "Why me?" "I hate my life; nothing ever goes right!" These beliefs are as deadly to our mental health as a daily diet of bacon is to our body! If this is you, the good news is that you will be able to feel much better soon.

What is a Mood?

Our moods (our basic state of mind) originate from the emotions and feelings that stem from our thoughts and beliefs about the moment we are in. These emotions or feelings can show up in obvious or subtle ways. The subtle emotions are often the ones that sneak up on us and make us moody. Normally, we tend to not notice or recognize background feelings because they are triggered by background thoughts and beliefs.

When you say, "I am not in a good mood," you refer to the background feelings of sorrow, unhappiness, unease, fear, or frustration. These feelings can manipulate your behavior because you are so unaware of them, and they can be the most dangerous. When someone barks, "Leave me alone; I am in a bad mood!" The person may as well be saying, "Something is pissing me off, and I have no freaking idea what it is!"

When this happens to you, you may be able to rattle off a list of problems, but it is actually the **thoughts/beliefs** about those problems that lead your mood down the dark tunnel. Unaware, you might suddenly snap at someone who asks a benign question or fly into a rage when the driver in front of you can't make up their mind. But the real reason you get angry may be that you were still thinking about the argument you had with your spouse that morning.

The amygdala is evaluating all thoughts and situations throughout the day, triggering both big and small warnings. We have learned throughout the years to dismiss the small warnings by simply pushing them away, not taking the time to shine the light of reality on them. So over the course of a day, these small ones gang up on us leaving us in a really crappy mood by the time dinner rolls around. Everything from feeling ignored in a meeting to having someone talk to you abruptly or having your boss give you less than his usual big smile can have your amygdala sounding the sirens.

Everyone is in a good mood the day before their long-awaited vacation begins or after their boss calls them aside to say he is very impressed with something they did. They will feel lighter and more cooperative with coworkers, all thanks to the serotonin release. Since serotonin makes you feel better than others (remember, that it's job), it also brings confidence, making you more open and agreeable. The opposite is true when you are brooding about something even as insignificant as your hair. Controlling these moods requires that you be able to trace them back to your various thoughts and beliefs, (both conscious and subconscious) that triggered the mood. It is there that you can dismantle the lies, replace them with facts, and feel better.

Time To Check In With Reality

Emotional moments are always a thought away. Real or imagined, any thought can cause an emotional upheaval and during that time, your thoughts *do not* represent an accurate picture of the truth. There are two ways an emotion is triggered. A thought may trigger an emotion, and the emotion makes us believe the thought was a fact. The second way is without words or thoughts; your limbic system (emotional area of your brain) evaluates a situation that does not seem favorable to you. In either case, the stress hormone cortisol is released, you feel bad, and then you try to find reasons that validate your emotion. We feel better when we know why something happens, even if we have to conjure up some plausible reason, and those reasons, are always are determined by our perspective. **Feeling bad is your "check reality light."** It means a thought is being allowed to stand as a fact. You can't allow that without confirming its reality first.

If any part of your body bothers you can assume that your belief is subtly affecting your mood. Most hate to admit this because it seems a bit shallow, but that is our reality. Evolution has hardwired it into our brain that to be desired ensures our survival, and to be desired means to have the right looks, money and sex appeal. Hence, our obsession with the rich and famous. By addressing any subtle beliefs about your looks under the scrutiny of facts, you can alleviate the cringe factor.

The Power of Our Physical Insecurity

Subtle beliefs such as "my hair looks so bad today," "I look so much older being bald," or "I wish my teeth weren't so crooked" can leave us with an underlying insecurity. If you are over 45 and are beginning to feel that your body is really showing it, you might be hearing more of these thoughts than ever before. It is like a problem that you can't put your finger on. For me, I have to remind myself to adjust my perspective to the facts. Another way to remedy these relentless thoughts is to allow nice compliments about your looks or body to really soak in. Don't play it down or dismiss it. Remind yourself that people are not saying something nice to you out of pity, even though your stupid amygdala may be telling you that.

The following examples show how a benign situation can trigger the alarm due to our perspective about the situation.

Thought / Situation	Perspective=Pain
Sitting home on the weekend.	My social life sucks, I never do anything.
Child seems in a mood	I feel like we are growing apart. Maybe I don't pay enough attention.
A coworker gets a raise	Why am I always ignored. No one ever sees how hard I try.
Driver pulls out in front of you	OMG! What a jerk I know he saw me and pulled out anyway!
Why haven't I heard from so-and-so?	They never call if they have something better to do. Why don't I have better friends?
Your cable bill arrives and has an added charge that you believe is wrong.	Those #$% think they can just rip people off! I can't afford to pay this: now I have to call and have a fight with them.
Coworker you thought you were pretty friendly with barely says "hi" in the hallway.	Wow, I thought we were friends. What did I do? Maybe some one bad-mouthed me.

 These situations trigger insecurity and frustration in you, but they are not the disaster your amygdala makes them out to be, screaming, "You might die if your boss doesn't notice you; you could die if you can't pay your bill!" So your brain contrives stories to both validate your anger and enrage it even more.

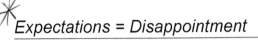
Expectations = Disappointment

Imagine being at home and something happens that really disappoints you. You are totally bummed. You put the TV on and what you see playing are all the times you have been let down or disappointed! You are stunned at you sit there watching when suddenly you can't believe how bad your life is. Well this is what happens in your mind whenever a situation arises that triggers any kind of negative reaction in you. Your memory jumps in and says, "wait a minute we have felt this before let me show you!" And it begins to replay similar past hurtful events. But why? To validate the fear, sadness, or anger, you are currently feeling. It's job is to recall past experiences of whatever your mind seems to be focused on in the moment. That is how you know what to do this time.

Well that is helpful when you are lost trying to remember what direction to go, or seeing something move in the bushes so you know whether to run or not. But other than that it can often be more harmful.

Up till now you have gone right along with these images allowing them to "rub salt in the wound" as they say. But this is another area where mindfulness will begin to be of tremendous benefit to you. As you are just learning you will miss this connection and go right along with it allowing the memories to validate your pain, but after practicing paying attention, you will catch what is going on before your head digs up every memory of having being treated unfairly.

Disappointment is a direct reflection of expectations. Expectations subtly sneak in, hanging around in the background. They are a result of you making subconscious decisions to expect an outcome of some sort. Becoming aware of these expectations early on is the key to avoiding these kinds of setbacks that can plague your mood all day long.

For example: after planning a weekend getaway with friends, you come down with the flu, which prevents you from going. You might consider that a legitimate disappointment, thinking to yourself, "Hey, you have every right to be upset here. I mean, was it too much to ask for a lousy weekend away?" Of course it wasn't; however, you will enlarge the disappointment if you choose to see it as something being taken from you or you being robbed of fun. That will throw you into a victim mentality, feeling sorry for yourself, with grand stories behind why you got sick, why life is unfair, and why these things always happen to you. These sad stories reside in your memory and come rushing in like witnesses to a crime to prove that life is treating you unfairly. With the emotions as fresh as the day the events took place, you will feel as though every bad thing that ever happened to you is happening *all over again!* It will leave you with a sense of hopelessness and anger. This reaction is often a learned behavior from your family. Watching other adults while you were growing up handle setbacks, failures, and disappointments sets the stage for how you will react. If all you ever heard was, "It never fails," "It figures," "Everything I try fails," and "Nothing is ever going to work out; why try?" Then you will have some beliefs to unlearn. Others are "Why is the world against me?" Or "Oh sure, it rains on my one day off." My personal favorite: "I'm hopeful, but I'm sure something will go wrong."

When things go wrong, it takes real effort to break the habit of weaving an entire story of injustice around a new disappointment. We want reasons to make sense of failures or disappointments, damn it! It makes the brain happy to know why things don't go right. Growing up, I would hear relatives say, "My ship will come in when I am at the airport." They declared it as though it were a badge of honor. Now I know why. Human beings find solace in feeling that we know our future. Good or bad, it gives our life a sense of predictability, making us feel somewhat more secure and stable, and that releases serotonin.

In fact, whenever you hear someone expounding on how bad life is and providing the proof of past experiences to anyone who will listen, understand that it is their way of feeling better about a crappy life…but more on this later.

Sometimes your memory just wants to support your self-pity. Maybe you see a car you would love to own. Subconsciously, you begin to feel a sense of frustration over not owning it. That frustration could be tied to a belief that life isn't fair; you work your butt off and still live paycheck to paycheck. Then your memory begins reminding you of all the things you want but can't afford. It is simply trying to help by validating your current emotion and beliefs. It will send you every memory of every disappointment and letdown, reinforcing your belief that life is unfair!

I remember sitting in church years ago and seeing a couple come in. They seemed to have a great relationship, and I was single. I noticed immediately that I began to feel sad and lonely. I tried to catch it because I was in church—not the place to be feeling sorry for myself. However, once those emotions were in play, everything I saw supported what I was feeling, which was feeling left out. "Why wasn't I sitting with friends? Why can't I meet someone?" In five minutes, I was thinking, "My life sucks; why do I even bother to go to church?"

The only reason this happened was that my amygdala enlisted the help of my memory to ensure I really knew just how crappy my life was. Not a damn thing changed in those five minutes. No epiphany, no new information, yet I suddenly felt I had a horrible life!

Our life does not have to be good for us to feel good about it, and it doesn't have to be bad for us to feel bad about it. We determine from the inside how we want to feel and proceed from there.

See if the following reactions sound familiar.

Disappointment	Memory-Perspective
Car broke down on the way home from work.	What a piece of junk! I should have never bought this car. This is going to cost a fortune again! I knew I couldn't trust that mechanic.
Sale item you have been waiting to buy is sold out.	This always happens I have the worst timing! I never get it right, and I always miss out.
You start your home computer just to be met with a blank screen.	Oh no, not again! I have bills to pay! I have no luck with computers!
Traffic tied up for miles on your way to run errands.	Not now! Every time I am in a rush this happens!
No parking space.	Not again! Now I have to pay for a space. I should have stayed home!
Your bank sends a letter saying you are overdrawn.	There is no way. They are just trying to get more fees. They are always squeezing more money out of me!
It rains on the one day you planned to be outside.	Really? Can't anything go my way? This happens every time! I swear, someone up there doesn't like me!

In a split second, your memory has scanned for similar experiences to validate your disappointment. Exaggerated perspectives are seen as infallible facts that fuel your anger. The reason is that once you are angry, your brain will not allow any information to get through that would <u>not</u> support your outrage. Without mindfulness you will buy into pretty much anything that it shows you.

Disarming Disappointments

Your brain doesn't care if you believe the story verbatim that it begins to show you. Your old programming thinks that sending you deeper into anger and frustration will fire you up, enabling you to make the changes required to fix the situation. Remember, that is a lie. We are not in the jungle with the lion anymore, and you don't need to fight, especially a disappointment. The mere concept is ridiculous, but we do it anyway, ranting on and on about our disappointment. We replay it over and over, embedding our anger and hurt into a new memory that we will now believe as fact. We never evaluate these memories that get brought up from our past; we just grab hold of them as though they were a friend coming to our aid.

This system is outdated. For example, if you suddenly feel lonely, your brain should tell you to call friends or go on a dating site, but that is not your memory's job. Instead it sends images of your last girlfriend or boyfriend to help motivate you to find someone new. But instead you think, "Wow, my ex must be thinking about me. Maybe I'm supposed to call him." Not!

Your brain likes to color things black and white. Similar to the statements I mentioned earlier that I heard growing up, you can see it in your memories: "This always...," "Nothing ever...," "I never...," and so on. This is also referred to as all-or-nothing thinking.

This role of memory when we need something can actually be dangerous for people fighting addictions. It is why breaking a habit of any kind often requires that they stay away from certain people, places, and things. When people start to have an emotion that they want to alleviate, the brain thinks it is helping by reminding them of what they did the last time they felt uncomfortable—which, for addicts, is usually a drug of some kind. The brain then releases dopamine in anticipation of the reward waiting on the other side of that drug use.

Before disappointment strikes, you must be vigilant in reminding yourself that setting your hopes on one particular event or occurrence is dangerous, unnecessary, and misleading. No event will make you happy forever! Everything is transient and passes. The most subtle ones are those we expect in the course of our day, such as getting to work on time, having no traffic, having the computer work, or having the bus be on time. All are setups for disappointment.

Now, of course, you don't want to expect bad things to happen, but you can't forget that life is unpredictable. If you have personal expectations, it will feel like a personal attack when things don't go your way, and you will fly into anger. Let me make this simple—**Don't cling to outcomes.** Before I leave the house, I remind myself that regardless of what my to-do list says, anything is possible today. Beginning your day with expectations is like shoving a ticking time bomb into your pocket. It is only a matter of time before it blows.

Do the following reactions sound familiar? *"Nice blinker, idiot!"* *"This stupid computer!"* *"Crap, it's only three o'clock."* *"Why is everyone driving like an ass?"* *"OMG, the Internet is so slow today!"*

These reactions are as helpful as throwing your shoe at the clouds because it is raining on your day off! You are personalizing all of these random events. Such reactions also cut you off from seeing just how amazing life is around you. Stay present to these ridiculous, hidden beliefs that will do their best to wreck your day before it starts. When you walk out the door, remind yourself that although you intend to do this or that, anything can happen. Doing this disarms your amygdala, which is always on the lookout for things not going according to your plan. So take your plan (expectation) off the table. Your amygdala is different from that of the next person; whatever you believe should or shouldn't happen is what it will try to protect, so only you can take down the beliefs/expectations that trigger it to begin with.

A research study found that Danish people are the happiest on earth, and the reason was that they have very modest expectations. They understand that life owes them nothing and that when things go well, it is a blessing. *They are living proof that keeping an attitude of appreciation and gratitude reduces stress and frustration.*

The Power of Your Core Energy

I would be remiss if I didn't mention another aspect of accepting negative beliefs about your life. Aside from making you feel miserable, negative energy can drive many of the events to and from your life. When you have a mind-set that expects bad things to happen, trust me—that is what will happen. The universe will deliver what you focus on and believe to be true about your life.

Several years ago, I began to understand that this principle is rooted in the science of quantum mechanics. I realized that my expectation of problems was not helping me in the least, so I began mediating each morning on new positive beliefs about how my life would go. There was an immediate shift in my finances—a $6,000 increase in two months. Although my prior beliefs had evolved due to real, factual patterns that kept happening to me, they were not moving my life forward, so I decided to develop new ones—and my life followed suit. This entailed a meditation on what I wanted in my life. As I focused on the details each morning, by the end of each thirty-minute session, my energy was bursting with excitement and anticipation about the good things that were coming. My entire energy force was radiating as if these things were already taking place. It is that energy force that can also alter your world.

The following exercise is an excellent source of help when you feel overwhelmed by shame, hurt, rejection, or fear. Which is all contrived perception. It will teach you to ascertain the facts in a given situation, not what you want to believe. On the left side, you write your thought or belief. On the right side, you write the fact that proves you are right. This fact has to be verifiable by an outsider, not an assumption, no matter what your history with that situation is. Almost every time, your facts will **disprove** what you believed about the situation, and seeing that will completely pull back the curtain of illusion and place your feet firmly back in reality.

COMPLETE WITH A RECENT EVENT OR LATER WHEN ONE TAKES PLACE.

Emotions	Facts
E.g. My boss has been acting weird. I feel like I am going to lose my job.	I have never been in trouble, my supervisor even said I did a good job on my report last month. I am always on time.

How often are you aware of why and when your moods change? Circle.

Very	1-3x a per day	No idea

Are you more aware of good moods or bad moods?

_____

Are you ever surprised at being in a good mood?

_____

Find someone at home or work to whom you can give a really nice compliment. Notice whether the person's mood seems to improve over the next hour or so. See if you felt anything as well. Describe below.

_____

_____

_____

_____

_____

_____

Mood Journal for a Week

Answer the questions below as you go through the week.

Give two examples of when your mood was lifted, even if the lift was subtle, because of something another person said or did.

_____

_____

_____

List five life events that can trigger a subtle good mood in you.

1._____

2._____

3._____

4. _____

5. _____

Did you notice being in a better mood after you accomplished tasks, whether at work or at home? List the tasks, big or small.

_____

_____

_____

_____

_____

_____

Give two examples of when your mood was down because of something another person said or did..

_____

_____

_____

List five life events that triggered a subtle bad mood in you.

1. _____

2. _____

3. _____

4. _____

5. _____

List five thoughts that have influenced your mood before you realized it.

1. _____

2. _____

3._____

4._____

5._____

After a day of lying around the house doing nothing, you can wind up feeling blah and empty, or in a crummy mood. Going a whole day with no purpose or accomplishments can drop your serotonin. It is a big no-no if you want to be happy. Describe such a day if you have had one.

_____

_____

How Do You Handle Disappointments

List the three negative beliefs you most commonly heard while growing up from those around you when things went wrong.

1._____

2._____

3._____

List the four negative comments about your life that you most commonly hear yourself saying or thinking (that you now realize are beliefs) when things go wrong.

1._____

2._____

3._____

4._____

See if you can recognize four of your own beliefs such as "life is unfair" that have made your disappointments feel like a personal assault.

1._____

2 _____

3 _____

4 _____

This week, write down three instances in which you realize you are letting a current disappointment color your feelings about your whole life, career, family, and future.

1 _____

2 _____

3 _____

List eight examples of when you had hidden expectations that you were unaware of until they did not come to pass and you became angry (anything from arriving at work on time to having a nice day with the family).

1 _____

2 _____

3 _____

4 _____

5 _____

6 _____

7 _____

8 _____

List six examples of when you have personalized a situation that was not personal from this week or from the past.

1 _____

2 _____

3 _____

4 _____

5 _____

6 _____

No need to do these exercises all at once. Refer to them at the end of each day until you are able to answer all of them.

_____

_____

_____

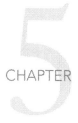

CHAPTER

Tantalizing Tantrums

In addition to being bad for the body, stress can stain our reputations as individuals with bad tempers or being a drama queen. Just *wanting* to be more calm and in control of our emotions is not enough; we have to be a little desperate, because many of us LOVE our Fury and will go down swinging when told we have to give it up if we really want happiness.

Letting go of your over reactive emotions might feel scary, counterintuitive, and even dangerous at first because you will feel like you're letting your guard down. I compare it to being asked to play a game of catch with your eyes closed. You want to have the confidence that the ball will land in the mitt, but you are also wincing because you know you could get hit in the face. That's what it feels like at first to let go of that protective shield of anger and frustration. We have all been there. Something happens, our fear turns into fury, and suddenly we feel like we are a force to be reckoned with—that somehow we will make whoever or whatever pay for messing with us. This is the philosophy we resort to in many cases; if we can't beat 'em, fight 'em anyway.

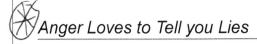

When something upsetting happens and you go along with that first rush of adrenaline, your brain will begin to send you every thought and memory possible to validate your anger and frustration and might even have pointing fingers. "It's their fault! Why does this keep happening? This is unfair!" So, within seconds, as the adrenaline begins to course through your veins, you are completely captivated. It will feel as if you are one with the emotion.

We find it very hard to separate from it in those first few minutes, but our interpretation of it is an illusion. We are not those emotions, and they are not accurate. They don't reflect reality as much as they reflect our overblown perspective of it in that moment.

When anger does overtake you, always remember that you are almost never upset for the reason you think you are. Only after you calm down will you see the truth, and it will almost always have its root in some kind of fear. I suggest to clients that when anger rises, they should stop and ask, "What am I afraid of right now?" Common fears are those of embarrassment, rejection, loss, and danger. Getting to that root will always put things in perspective.

When you get upset, your brain knows that you need something at that moment, so you may experience a hundred images in seconds, giving rise to anger, frustration, self-pity, and loneliness that support and validate your current belief about the situation. This can happen quickly especially when you are disappointed by someone close to you. The next time someone does something to upset you, see if you can spot how many "blaming" memories flood in to validate your outrage toward this person. You will have to be fast because the memories will be there in under a second yelling, "Pick me! Hey, over here! I can prove he did that on purpose. I can show you that she doesn't really care." Next thing you know, you become angrier at the person than the situation warrants, and when pressed for a reason, you will probably bark, "Because you always do this!" Your brain is programmed to ignore any information that would disprove your violated feelings. It does this to protect you.

We are just as hard on ourselves when we make mistakes, wondering, "Just how many freaking times do I have to forget my cell phone to figure out a better system?" Very often a current frustration is further fueled by a past experience. I have had plenty of clients who report hearing one of their parents voices in their head chastising them for their screw up. For example, forgetting your cell phone triggers the memory of your parents yelling at you for being an airhead thirty years ago. So there you are, ready to berate yourself and carry on the pattern.

Deciding to not throw tantrums is one of the hardest obstacles to overcome if that is your pattern, but it is easier when you reconcile how silly it is and what a false sense of protection it gives. Thankfully, even a little progress in this area will yield big results. When you feel rattled, just taking a long breath at the beginning of the upheaval will change your chemistry enough for you to stay present. You need to remind yourself that you are not going to die from this or that, and you need to place the blame where it really belongs—with that lizard brain of yours. Please don't dismiss the small steps you make in this area; they are bigger than you think and should be celebrated.

How Feeling Bad, Can Feel So Good

If negative feelings feel so terrible to us, we might wonder why we all aren't optimists, seeing the world through rose-colored glasses. The truth is, we don't need to do that because the brain can enjoy feeling bad. Our lives, or sections of it at least, are uncertain to some extent, and any kind of uncertainty is the enemy of a happy brain. Being unsure reduces your sense of safety and security, leaving you feeling vulnerable because your serotonin took a dip.

Bosses often make the big mistake of allowing employees to feel that their jobs are not secure, assuming this insecurity will motivate them to work harder. When in fact, it makes them much less productive because they live in fear and crisis mode.

When uncertainty has you rattled, you may engage in any of the following behaviors to increase some brain chemicals, but the benefits are short-lived. If you complain to other coworkers about how bad your company or boss is, those who agree with you will make you feel safer and more connected because of serotonin and oxytocin. If you put the government or world leaders down, predicting doom and gloom, you make the world feel predictable, releasing some serotonin. Even making false predictions about the future will make you feel superior. If you like to get fired up and debate or argue about life events, you will release dopamine. Misery doesn't just love company; it needs it! It allows us to crawl on our knees, bleeding and bruised, side by side, and feel that it's us against them...whoever "them" is at the time. Next time you are waiting in line in a public place, see how long it takes for someone to make eye contact with you and roll their eyes, as if to say, "Do you believe this?"Eventually someone else might either speak up with sarcasm or make some kind of disgruntled noise, and then for a moment or two you will all feel better.

Have you ever made eye contact with someone to get them to agree with your frustration only to have them dismiss you like it's no big deal? Remember, if others don't validate your emotions, serotonin can dip because your amygdala starts the warning bells: "How dare you ignore this blatant waste of our time? What is wrong with you; are you telling me you don't see this?"

Such scenarios are always around the next corner. These are our primal instincts when we are violated or frustrated: first see who around us is on our side. A dog's primal instinct when he is unsure around another dog is to sniff the other dog's butt. At least we have evolved to look for signs above the waistline.

Your Amygdala Needs Drama Rehab!

With all of the stress and drama you are dealing with during the day, it is important to mention the unyielding determination of your amygdala to stress you out at night as well. It is sooooo addicted to stress and drama that some nights, like an addict, it will reach for one more hit right before bed. Does this sound familiar?

Your head hits the pillow and you begin having a heated one-sided discussion with that coworker, child, or spouse, and although this is happening only in your head, you get as angry and upset as if it were happening in real life, with all the same harmful chemicals in play. (My personal favorite is rehashing a situation from childhood or with someone who isn't even in my life anymore.) Talk about insane behavior! Over and over in your head, you will make your point, chasing some sort of elusive validation like a dog chasing his tail. Before you know it, you're tossing and turning and can't sleep.

For others, fears of your loved ones being in danger take over. If you are a parent you know this all too well and mothers are especially good at it. As we toss and turn witnessing this horror movie of our own making, we search for any reliable gut feeling or sense that we are correct in our fears. As if knowing something bad was coming would allow us to prevent it anyway. Take it from an over protective aunt who has had her share of sleepless nights *for no reason*, if you think your fears have any basis then pray. At least I feel like someone with more wisdom and power is responsible now. Oh sure were their dangers at some point, yes but never affiliated with a particular night of tossing and turning. So after all the stress one day can hand you, you climb into bed exhausted and your brain hops back on the Worry-Go-Round.

Some of us start our day playing this make-believe game with our adversaries in our bathroom while we are getting ready for work! Who hasn't mentally told someone off while getting ready in the morning? By time you leave the house, you are ready to explode and have put yourself in a horrible mood. You need to be alert for these autopilot moments. You have to catch them quickly because once cortisol is released, it takes about thirty minutes to subside. You might as well hang a **WARNING** sign around your neck for a half hour. And there you have it: You are in a "mood" and have no idea how you got there. Not to mention you have now shortened your fuse and anything could ignite it.

Are You Known for Overreacting?

Has anyone ever told you that you worry too much? If so, do you agree?

_____

Are you known for having a bad temper?

_____

Who have you hurt by blowing up?

_____

_____

Describe two situations in which you have embarrassed yourself by blowing up.

1._____

_____

_____

2._____

_____

_____

Do you notice how empowered or strong you feel while you are blowing off steam?

_____

_____

_____

Letting go of this reaction can make you feel vulnerable. Describe an example of what it felt like trying to control your rage. What thoughts went through your head?

_____

_____

Monologues

How often do you have these monologue arguments? (Circle)

1-3 x per month   **More than 5x per month**

Where do you do it the most? (Circle)

In bed   In the shower   While driving

Getting ready in the morning

List the types of situations you rehash from the day, from your past, and in preparation of a future situation.

Day

_____

_____

_____

_____

_____

Past

_____

_____

_____

_____

_____

Preparation for the future

_____

_____

_____

_____

Do you ever try to stop yourself once you realize you are getting upset?

_____

How difficult is that?

_____

List the four people you most often do this with in your head.

1. _____

2. _____

3. _____

4. _____

List two instances this week when you have tried to catch these auto pilot moments. Were you able to stop before you were too upset? Describe below.

1. _____

_____

2. _____

_____

_____

CHAPTER

Who's In Charge Here?

HAVE YOU EVER BEEN IN A STORE AND SUDDENLY HEARD THE BLOOD CURDLING SCREAMS OF A TODDLER? If you are like me, after about 30 seconds you are wondering when the heck the parent is going to calm his child down.

Meanwhile, in many cases, the parents act as if they barely notice. It's because they know they can't reason with their child at that point, and such is the case for adults when under the control of their lizard brain. As a chemical fire storm transpires in our brain, all common sense is put on hold, we behave like that child; act out and think unreasonably.

The newest part of our brain the prefrontal cortex, ideally should enable us to over ride our lizard brain and be calm and reasonable in the face of problems and disappointments. However, that takes maturity and our brains aren't even fully developed until we are about twenty-seven years old. By that time we are pretty adept at allowing our rage and frustration to over take us. This prefrontal cortex is our awareness system; it is where we decide, plan, and make responsible choices. I referred to it earlier as our "head office" This is what gives us the capacity to think out into the future, back into the past and then evaluate both to make sense of the present.

Right now the one who is in charge of your behavior/feeling center is your *back office*, not your newer reasonable thinking *front office* as you might hope. Initially this older brain has most of the control in how you are influenced; it draws conclusions about people you don't really know, deems others dumb or ignorant before you have even one conversation with them, and dislikes or champions people through beliefs you don't even know you have. It will believe a total stranger and refute your friends based on a gut feeling instead of information, it will join a team of people you don't know, and defend causes you know very little about. It is where your beliefs and opinions are protected to the death. In short this is your ego personified.

In social situations, specifically, it is very important to be aware of your own thoughts; otherwise, your subconscious can very subtly have you drawing a biased conclusion about people without you even knowing it. This is how prejudices, judgments, and attitudes begin to form. Never dismiss how crafty your brain can be once it has made a preconceived judgment about someone because it will look for every possible behavior and comment to reinforce your beliefs—and trust me, it will find them. Like I mentioned in chapter one, your brain is programmed to see and hear what it needs in order to reinforce any belief it wants to protect.

If you have ever been on the receiving end of prejudice, it's confusing and hurtful. Nothing you do can bridge this chasm of mistrust and dislike because they are totally unaware of why they have drawn this conclusion about you. Some people may describe it as a gut feeling they can't really explain, but they will stand by it until a mountain of opposing proof shows up—and even then some still won't change their opinion.

I remember spending one summer in the company of a new group of people; all of them seemed warm and genuine except one woman. I tried to connect, but she wanted nothing to do with me. One day I finally told a close friend who had known this woman for years what I had noticed. She smiled and said, "Oh, I know why; you are a dead ringer for the woman her husband had an affair with and eventually left her for." Ahh, there it was. This woman was completely controlled by an experience from five years ago and had no idea that she was allowing it to drive her feelings and perception about a virtual stranger! Short of my undergoing plastic surgery or an extreme makeover, our friendship did not stand a chance. Although I admit that I was tempted to explain it to her, but I decided to move on. Contemplate how powerful a tool this is and you will quickly realize how unconscious many of your actions and decisions are. It is downright scary.

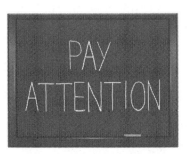

However, we finally have a way to expose all of these "back office politics". The portal by which we can now **listen** to what is happening in our subconscious is through our **prefrontal cortex**. Imagine your "head office" finally taking charge and saying, "Nothing happens without us being made aware of it first!" No special equipment required. All you need is the very same skill that teachers tried to get us to practice when we were children. It was two words we heard almost every day: **"Pay attention!"** Unfortunately, even as adults we are no better at this and in many cases worse.

Paying attention is the practice of single-minded focus, meaning we learn to be fully aware of the here and now, not off in the future or in the past. This allows us to finally know what the other part of our brain is thinking, so our emotions are not tossed about all day like a boat without an anchor. If you were a company today would be the day to put up a new sign that says, UNDER NEW MANAGEMENT.

The Cause of Absentmindedness

Although our prefrontal cortex is our head office, the back office, lizard brain has been here longer, so it thinks it has seniority so to speak. It is up to you to teach the front office to exercise its authority. You do that by training it to pay attention. No more drifting, no more casual focus. In order to be in charge it has to know what is coming out of the back office. When we don't we are like robots so lost in incessant thinking that we can drive home and have no idea how we got there, walk into rooms and have no clue why, and lose our keys, wallets, and purses all because our minds are convinced that the noise going on in our heads is more important than what is happening around us.

About a decade ago, neuroscience began probing the cause of this excessive mind wandering, and it seems to be the default state the mind goes to whenever we lose interest in what we are doing or become tired. And now thanks to all of our modern marvels we now have the attention span of eight seconds, so now we are almost never here in the moment! The purpose of this wandering state seems to be so we can decide whether our reaction to our spouse this morning was warranted. However, this program is broken, so instead of thinking through the issues at hand and drawing helpful, insightful conclusions, we ruminate repeatedly over situations, conversations, and even a single sentence said to us ad nauseam.

This reptilian brain of yours, is the seat of your unconscious and can process more than 200,000 bits of info per second! That is a lot of processing power. So about every eight seconds, or whenever you get bored it takes over grabbing memories from your past, speculating on your future, and scanning your environment for danger, which could mean just a dirty look. This so constant that it becomes an energy you can actually feel in your physical body, like an undercurrent of anxiety or worry, even though you may not be aware of it. Being distracted by all this internal noise can result in your moving about restlessly, recklessly, dropping things, or even being a klutz. The most common symptom, though, is that it leaves you absentminded and forgetful.

Although all of this processing is happening under the surface it triggers automatic speculations and fears, that eventually make their way up to our front office where you can become aware of them as moods, attitudes and beliefs. Once your front office is in charge it will address these concerns or fears with facts. At first glance, I realize that speculating on future problems may seem helpful and even responsible; however, you will almost never predict anything close to what actually happens. In addition, most of the time your brain will minimize the resources you have to handle a problem and exaggerate possible outcomes, so instead of feeling better prepared, you wind up feeling doomed.

You need to set aside time to review the issues at hand and make plans and set goals, but then you must let them go. That allows your subconscious to dig in and pull out the best answers. You know, the ones that come to you in the shower or in your sleep. That is the genius of your subconscious, but that will not happen if your mind is engulfed in fear, holding onto the problem, rehashing the same information. Remember that your brain does not know the difference between real or imagined, and 85 percent of the time, it will imagine the worst. Again, we are stuck on the *Worry-Go-Round*™.

I love the car commercial on TV that illustrates this absentmindedness so well. The driver is going over in his head everything on his plate for the day, and in so doing he almost has three collisions. Fortunately, his pricey car's technology saves the day by stopping him before he crosses into the other lane and hits the other cars.

Well, that car may have kept him safe physically, but it did nothing to protect his emotions, which were dragged all over as his mind raced from one potential problem to another. There is a time for reflection, but it needs to be a deliberate decision on our part. We can't just allow the mind to wander off by itself, getting into any trouble it can find. Although, we come hardwired to do just that, once your front office is in charge—you will break this formidable habit.

Like a dog that knows how to be attentive when a sound suddenly breaks the night silence, so it is with most of us. We can concentrate when something of interest grabs our attention, but now we need to learn to stay in that place of focused attention. We

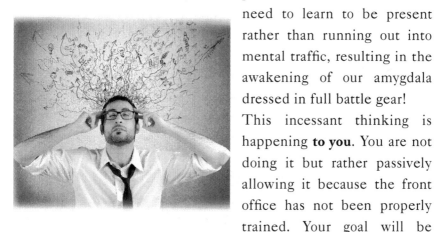

need to learn to be present rather than running out into mental traffic, resulting in the awakening of our amygdala dressed in full battle gear! This incessant thinking is happening **to you**. You are not doing it but rather passively allowing it because the front office has not been properly trained. Your goal will be to disassociate with these passing thoughts, thereby distancing yourself from any emotion they trigger. You learn to observe them not be dragged around by them. If you have ever tried to focus your attention during a lecture, meeting, or while in church I am sure you noticed your untrained mind chasing every passing thought, just like a dog trying to absorb every scent as he sticks his head out of the car window. Any thought that makes you feel threatened, afraid, concerned, annoyed, frustrated, or demeaned—and of course, on the other spectrum, heroic, amazing, smart, creative, interesting, and funny—will all be a distraction. This is a tantalizing smörgåsbord for the mind, either happily keeping you from the reality of a bad day or burying you further in despair. Being tossed about all day at the mercy of whatever those seventy thousand thoughts want to say will leave you at the end of every day the way you began it—frustrated, upset, and tired.

Single Minded Attention

Being focused on what is happening right here and now allows for greater emotional tolerance when something does happen that you did not expect, such as traffic, no parking space, or lost

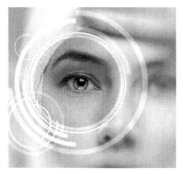

keys. You will notice these issues won't fluster you the way they did before. Let me explain one reason why.

None of us likes to be interrupted. If we're reading, writing, talking, or watching TV, interruptions disrupt our flow and cause a slight annoyance. Well, in the course of the average day, the mind is often racing back and forth

thinking about everything except the now. So when something happens in the now, like you spill some milk, it's an interruption to your brain. Your brain has to stop its racing and focus on the here and now. You know this is happening when you hear yourself bark, "Damn it!" However, when you are totally present, you will notice almost zero frustration because you are already "here" nothing catches you off guard. Your focus on the present causes you to see things with an interest and slight fascination similar to that of a wide-eyed child so that almost anything that happens just draws more interest. I have to say that of all the benefits this one is my personal favorite. I was cleaning the kitchen one day staying very present when I lifted the salt shaker and the bottom fell out. I stopped moving and found myself staring at it taking in what just happened. No swearing, zero frustration. That is when I realized this sense of intense interest. I felt like the world stopped spinning and nothing else mattered. Until you experience this you can't really understand the sense of utter freedom from reaction and emotion. This is the road to peace and happiness. This is what will give you lasting peace of mind. Single-minded attention is the point and focus of most meditation and mindfulness practices.

Now at first glance stopping this ruminating might seem to require control, but what it really takes is *trust* and *courage*. It will feel very unnerving to stop peering into the future for threats, dangers, and possible mishaps. However, when you ignore even a few minutes down the road, you will begin to feel that happiness and peace you so deserve. *Learn the rules: allowing your brain to go into the future unattended will bring anxiety, and allowing it to drift casually into the past will make you mad/sad. Remember, you hold the leash!*

Staying in the present moment, and not allowing your mind to consider any possible problems even ten minutes down the road is a little like setting a clock ahead by ten minutes. Maybe you have done this yourself to ensure you get somewhere on time. You have to make a choice to follow the time on the clock rather than the actual time. You know both pieces of information, but you choose to take the clock at face value. Doing that takes trust because it will feel like you are letting your guard down, but that is only an illusion. If your mind isn't in this moment, the moment isn't worth living. *It's your focus and attention that give it value.*

Aside from any underlying mental conditions Your goal is to never have a mood lower than a six on a scale of one to ten. By doing the practices in this book, you will start to see an increase in your mood level. When you start to feel upset, you will be able to say, "Wait, this is a false alarm; I don't have to go along with this."

Eckart Tolle, a popular spiritual leader, teaches people how to stay in the present moment without actually practicing meditation. However, when people are initially learning to slow down their mind, it is helpful to begin such a practice in a controlled environment, like with meditation.

I learned to stay in the present in a mere five days while on vacation reading Eckart Tolle's book A New Heaven and a New Earth. Vacation was the perfect setting to be calm and practice for ten days straight. By day three, I was already feeling a totally different vibe in my focus, and by day five, I was walking around fascinated by the intense focus I could give to everything that crossed my path. Worry and fears had dropped away because the present moment was the only thing that seemed real to me.

Around the eighteenth day, I was driving my car totally engrossed in the moment when I suddenly had a sense of boredom. That's right, boredom! There had been no panic, drama, anger, or frustration for seventeen days, and part of me seemed to be missing that stupid energy. Well, back then, the step I was missing was *taking in the good*. I didn't understand that the second part to this process was allowing myself to feel every wonderful feeling of security, safety, and love from those around me, allowing that to translate into appreciation and gratitude. I did not at that point understand that my amygdala was still looking for problems and that my brain was still very invested in fighting for my survival. Being chill and letting most things handle themselves until my action was required was not a neural pattern yet.

So I was driving my car, feeling as though I had been safe indoors from inclement weather, when I felt like I just had to poke my head out and see how things were coming along down the road. In essence, I started thinking and worrying about things before there was any reason to do so. Just being safe and feeling good was foreign to my mind, and being this calm began to send signals that something was amiss. So down the road I went, assuring myself that I could both look for problems and still maintain my new calmness. Within an hour, I was getting aggravated. **The absence of stress will never be enough, we need to feel the good.** *Your brain is never neutral it has to be engaged somewhere and you choose where that is!*

On days when you are running around trying to cram three days of errands into one, life may jump up and slap you—it always does eventually—and when it does you will find your footing again by simply adjusting your perspective and refocusing careful attention to the moment at hand. Sometimes I stop, close my eyes, take a deep breath, and just feel my feet on the floor. That reels my thinking and emotions in quickly. Another tool I use if I am home is I stand on a balance disc . This works even under extreme emotion. It is a round inflated disc you stand on. By closing your eyes and trying to maintain balance you immediately stop all other thoughts as all your attention is drawn to maintaining your balance. See my website for more details www.shariespironhi.com.

When people first begin practicing this present awareness, they often report sudden sensations pleasant, peaceful feelings just arising. You will see how your mind really loves focusing on only one thing at a time, it is like giving it a spa day. All that mental chatter is exhausting. Remember the disabled kids I talked about in the beginning of the book? Well, I have since discovered another reason for their positive demeanor is in part a result of their focusing all of their attention and energy on trying to move one limb at a time, and their brains are quite happy doing just that—one thing at one time.

Your Goal is This Moment —Not The Task

Most of us approach our list of tasks for the day as a challenge. Each task we can check off sends a shot of serotonin, making us feel accomplished.

However, no task is ever your goal; rather, your goal is to give the utmost careful attention to each moment. The present moment is not an obstacle to get past so you can get to the "next thing" No step you take can be seen as just a means to accomplishing the task; if it is, then most tasks will feel empty with no purpose until the very end when you check them off your "to do list" Why wait until the end of your task to get that serotonin when you can have it throughout the whole process? You will find purpose in each moment when you recognize that each step you take toward a task is in itself the purpose. This understanding is not complex, but it is the antithesis of how we think normally; Once you understand this fact your whole life will begin to feel different.

A great place to start this practice is while cooking a meal because it is often a place where we pay little attention. You set your intention to relish the purpose in each step or movement required to create that meal. You don't diminish the steps it takes to make the dinner and revel only in eating the dinner; rather, you keep your full attention focused on every physical movement that each moment requires. This exercise by itself will transform your mind in just days. As you walk into the kitchen, your footsteps are all that you pay attention to. As you reach down for a pot, that is the only thing you are thinking about. As you place it on the stove and turn the burner on, you observe your own movement with absolute focus. Sound silly? You won't believe how your mind calms down.

The degree to which the present moment holds your attention is the degree of success you will have in the next moment.

You will also be amazed at the natural sense of appreciation you can cultivate when you take your time like this. This understanding has been the entire point of practices such as yoga and Tai Chi for hundreds of years. The bliss people report experiencing when they only focus on the now is in part due to their cortisol levels dropping as their attention is on the here and now and not looking for the next thing that can go wrong. Their mind begins to experience a sense of calm security. (In the next chapter there will be exercises for this)

This moment is all you are responsible for, and you will find that most of your so-called problems never seem to quite make it into "this moment". Right now, close your eyes and recognize that this very moment is just fine; you are safe, have access to water and food, have a roof over your head, and are not in crisis. Once you get used to accepting each moment at face value, you will see a ton of things to smile and feel good about. We will cover more about that in the next chapter.

The more often you do this, the more DOS (dopamine, oxytocin, serotonin) are released into your synapse, moving your natural state of mind toward appreciation and gratitude, which will translate into a state of well-being. This is where the science meets the road. And, yes, for now your biased brain will still fight to focus on the negative because doing so is a very ingrained pattern, but in only a couple of weeks, the rewiring will begin. Then it will become more natural for you to be happier more often and to worry less.

Staying Present

A great way to know if your mind has slipped away from the now is to note whether you are bored, if there is tension in your muscles, or if you are doing something with an unnecessary intensity. For example, as you wash dishes, notice if you feel any intensity, speed, or tension in your muscles. You will notice the muscle tension most often while doing mindless activities such as preparing dinner, washing your hands, cleaning something, or even putting away groceries. I tend to do it most while preparing something to eat. It could be because I always wait till I am starving, but I remind myself to breathe and feel what is going on in my muscles.

When beginning a mindless activity, pause and notice what your body feels like. If it is brimming with intensity, notice that just by taking a moment to focus on it, your body and mind will slow back down. If you continue to pause intermittently to take note of your body's energies, you might be amazed at how fast the energy returns to a state of tension even after just one minute. If you are angry, you may feel empowered by this kind of energy. You may feel it will help you to finish your task more efficiently. It doesn't, however, because the energy is there without a focused mind to make the most of it. Being still and breathing deeply will cause a physiological alteration that can bring a calm to almost any moment.

RULE: Be **mindful** when you are doing something **mindless**.

Our Furry Friends Are Great Role Models

Our furry friends are great role models. Your golden retriever puppy is happy to put aside the toy he is disemboweling and clear his schedule to take a walk with you. He doesn't stress about how he is going to finish shredding the toy or think about how a walk might interfere with his existing plan to move on to the rawhide bone. Animals know how to live in the present moment, which is why they are eager to share such warmth with you.

It is simply a matter of what you really want in life, how happy you want to be, and the commitment you want to make. As with sticking with the gym or a diet, you have to give it time to transcend into a lifestyle. This rule does not bend: *joy can be experienced only in the present, not in the future or past.* So if joy is what you really want in life, why go looking in places where it will never be found. Joy is a bit different than happiness or calm it is almost divine but it evolves from moments of calm and happiness.

Life is one hell of a challenge; we do not need to make it any harder or more disappointing. However, keep in mind that some people like to invite drama into their lives, as they crave the madness and emotional mess to feel alive, although they will deny this emphatically. We all know people like that. We all have blind spots to varying degrees that can only be cleared by impeccable objectivity, or the help of a good friend who can point it out to us.

Time to Slow Down

Exercise One: Do at Home

Prepare yourself a cup of your favorite beverage. Go from sitting and reading this book to placing it down, standing up, and taking your first step and then another with total concentration. Find your cup or mug, and continue each step with absolute attention until your beverage is brewing or ready to drink. Then answer the questions below.

Did you notice that you physically slowed down so you could pay attention to each move?

_____

_____

Were you relaxed or tense while trying to concentrate?

_____

_____

Did it feel more natural as you went along?

_____

_____

Did you get frustrated or annoyed?

_____

Did you notice things you don't normally notice in the process? If so what?

_____

Exercise Two: Do at Home

Make yourself a simple snack. Again, put this book down, stand, and begin walking into your kitchen. Let no movement go unnoticed. Even if you are just turning your body to reach for something, notice each aspect of the movement. No need to study it; just observe with great attention as if you were moving your body for the first time.

Was it more natural this time?

_____

Did you feel frustrated at any point?

_____

What did you notice about your thinking?

_____

_____

_____

_____

Did anything happen to pull you out of this attentive mode? Explain:

_____

_____

Circle your overall feeling when done.
RELAXED   TENSE   SAME   Other_____

Practice this exercise throughout your day with things that you normally do mindlessly, such as showering, shaving, brushing your teeth, making your bed, vacuuming, driving, putting on make-up, or preparing for bed.

CHAPTER

7

Mindfulness/Meditation

Mindfulness is sometimes referred to as a technology of sorts because its effects are measurable; but the best part is you don't have to believe in it to see results. It just works. It has been proven to do the following:

- **Increase focus and concentration**
- **Reduce emotional reactivity**
- **Reduce stress**
- **Improve memory**
- **Enhance empathy**
- **Increase cognitive flexibility**
- **Lower sensitivity to pain**

I don't know about you, but I would do almost anything to get all of these benefits at once! This is a vast subject that could fill 10 giant books but suffice it to say that you learn it simply by doing it. There is no other practice out there that can give you this kind of mental and emotional enhancement, producing the fastest changes in your brain and your life. So just do it!

A simple mindfulness practice every morning, if only for one to five minutes, is all it takes to start. Before you tell me you can't do that because your mind wanders, know that such an argument is like saying you can't go to a gym because you are out of shape. You do this to gain control over the wandering! Now don't get all wigged out about this. If you are someone who has been avoiding this kind of practice, but are still unhappy. Maybe it's time to give it a try. I promise there is no sitting cross-legged, no "ohm-ing," and no trying to stop your mind from thinking! Thinking is what your mind does. You are going to learn to steer the thinking. The act of mindfulness or meditation is simply maintaining a pure awareness that allows you to become extremely aware of each thought going through your mind, that is often produced from your subconscious. Without doing this you will have no idea what is traveling through your mind in nanoseconds.

Teaching your brain to develop this new state of awareness is exactly like going to the gym for your body. Physical exercise takes some effort and discipline at first, but after about two months, you notice your body beginning to change. Similar will be your journey with meditation. You schedule your time each morning, and although time is precious, you realize that your well-being is, too. The first few weeks, you will feel awkward, uncertain if you are doing it right and unsure what difference you are even looking for. But as with the gym, you only have to do one thing, and that is show up and practice each morning. You have never studied your own mind before, it's only the most complicated, brilliant mechanism known to mankind. So don't assume it should be easy to control it for even one minute. If it were, everyone would be doing it! This practice is not an option but an imperative to retrain your brain to focus on all the good around you. I have no doubt that we will look back over history in fifty years or so and laugh at how we worked to build our bodies way before we ever tried to build our minds. OK, are you pumped?

One way—and there are many ways of teaching yourself to pay attention—is to train your mind to listen or just sit and feel your feet on the floor. Putting together thirty seconds of total concentration without allowing your mind to drift away will begin to rewire your mind; literally, areas of your brain will begin to reorganize. According to the National Center for Biotechnology Information, US National Library of Medicine, humans have an attention span of only eight seconds (goldfish have an attention span of nine seconds). I encourage the listening technique because it compels us to quiet the inner chatter, which can be the greatest obstacle in the beginning of this training. It also develops a skill that can help us function better in every facet of life.

Right from your first session, you will notice endless streams of thought that are controlling, motivating, inspiring, and deflating you, but in a couple of months you will stop being swept away by them. Mindfulness is not new, but it has really exploded over the past ten years, and there are tons of books out there for you to explore further. You can be your worst critic, so attempting a mindfulness/meditation practice on a day when your mind is overactive can be a real challenge. This is all part of the journey. If you were able to focus all your attention at this point, you would miss out on a crucial step. It is here, when your mind is racing all over, that you will learn the most about your negativity bias and your deep-seated beliefs. You will notice all the exaggerated thoughts and patterns of anger, blame, unforgiveness, and fear that have been controlling your behavior for years. Don't be overwhelmed; it is in the seeing of them that you will be able to cut their strings.

Keep a journal and see if you can pinpoint how and when your thought patterns affect your reactions or mood during the day. Your mind is not under your control yet. Every negative thought you have, even one such as "*I have to learn this mindfulness right now!"* will trigger your brain's life-or-death panic button. Relax; don't feed into that lie. This is a practice, like that of learning a musical instrument. You will have days in which you can really feel the progress and others when it feels like nothing is happening. Like a toddler learning to walk for the first time, embrace the learning curve and see it as an adventure. You will notice that on the days when you are able to focus for a long period, you will feel empowered and have a sense of calm throughout your day. Then the very next day, it might seem as though you took amphetamines before your practice, and you will feel like you are wasting your time. Just hang in there; your mind is not used to being on a leash. It will fight to visit old memories one minute and then worry about your future the next. That is the wiring you are breaking down. Every time you catch yourself being dragged off by erroneous thoughts and you stop to bring your attention back to the present moment, you are dismantling the old wiring system and instituting a new one!

At the end of this chapter there are practices for you to try as well as at the back of this book there is a more formal step-by-step description of how to begin.

In the exercise below, you will begin to notice the cues that set off your amygdala and the most common bunny trails your mind likes to revisit time and time again that usually leave you upset, angry, or frustrated. Each time you notice you are stuck in an old thought pattern, you will now have a chance to change the station. Breathe, feel your feet on the ground, and focus on the now, seeing all of the positive goodness around you. And always remind yourself that it is *your right to be happy*, not some gift you have to wait for life to give you.

The following practices, along with taking in the good, will change your life as you learn to hear all of the thoughts going through your head in the course of your day. You will soon see that the *root of all your emotional pain is 90 percent thoughts and mental chatter.* Strive for one minute of complete focused attention. Each week, add another thirty seconds. When your mind drifts, start over until you complete the amount of time you are trying for.

Three Mindful Practices

Practice 1

Sit upright in a comfortable chair, eyes closed. Take five long inhalations, and exhale twice as slowly as you inhale, if possible. Afterward, place the tip of your tongue underneath your two front teeth. Just as this prevents you from talking, it sends a signal to your brain to stop the mental chatter. Allow your eyes to gently gaze upward into your forehead. This helps raise alpha brain waves that settle your mind. Begin listening to any sounds outside of yourself, such as birds, the wind or rain, wind chimes, or even just the silence. This is not a casual attention; rather, it is a focused attention as you pick just one sound to listen for, as if you were listening for someone to whisper your name. Your first goal is to do this for thirty seconds without being distracted by passing thoughts. As you do notice thoughts, you will just let them drift by like clouds in the sky by immediately focusing your attention on your body for tension and consciously relaxing it. Every thought you notice is to trigger your attention back to the sound. Do not be harsh with yourself when thoughts arise. Thinking about other things is what your brain is used to doing. Just continue to listen for outside sounds. If you find yourself carried away momentarily following a thought, even for four or five seconds, begin your thirty seconds over again. If using sound is not comfortable for you, then by all means simply focus on your breath, just noticing the slow, deliberate inhale and exhale. **After your first attempt, applaud yourself! Many won't even attempt what you just did.**

Practice 2

Use this practice when your mind is wandering so much that you are getting more frustrated than relaxed. This will take five minutes. Take five long inhalations, and exhale twice as slowly as you inhale. Sit upright and just listen to your breath or another sound. Then wait thirty seconds and check your shoulders, back, and arms for tension. You will notice how your body is reacting to all the thoughts racing through your head even as you try to sit calmly. As you notice tension, just relax your shoulders, arms, lower back, or whatever part of your body is reacting. Do this until you can go one minute without tensing up.

It will amaze you how quickly your body will tense up again. Doing this each morning will help you remember to check your body during the day for this tension buildup. Once you are able complete one minute straight for three consecutive days, try going to two minutes with the same process. If your mind wanders, start over until you complete two minutes.

The Internet has many types of guided meditations for you to experiment with, and there are FREE down loadable meditation links on my website. Everyone is different. For me, using guided meditations that take me through my entire body don't seem to allow me to enter into any state of real stillness. That could be because such a technique employs the mind's various regions by requiring that it pay attention to various parts of the body. However, other guided meditations that just talk every few minutes and remind me to focus have been just right for me.

Practice 3: (For a Really Busy Brain)

If you are feeling hyper and distracted, try this. Sit in a place in the room where you have never sat before, a place that will give you a completely new angle on the room (that may mean on the floor). Sit with your eyes closed, take three deep breaths, and try to imagine you are in a dream. Then open your eyes and slowly look around the room from this new perspective. Try to recapture the feeling you have when dreaming, when nothing is in your mind but what you are seeing. Try to soak in everything with deliberate attention as if this were the most important dream you ever had, trying to memorize each detail. Do this for one minute without letting your mind think about what you are seeing. No cleaning the cobwebs you might spot—just sit and observe.

Sitting in a different area in a room can be very helpful because whenever you see or experience something new, your brain creates new neurons for learning. Those new neurons can be very helpful in bringing a heightened awareness to a situation, and with that awareness comes a focused calm. This is why vacations are so powerful. Your brain is flush with new neurons, bringing you into a state of calm, focused attention.

BEGINNING YOUR DAILY MEDIATION/MINDFULNESS PRACTICE

Day 1

If you found that your mind kept bouncing all over (99 percent will), did you notice any one prevalent thought? If so, which one?

_____

Was it a problem, a memory, or a recurring dialogue with another person?

_____

How many times did you have to start over?_____

Did you let yourself get frustrated over your mind wandering?_____

Describe your first attempt here. Was it harder or easier than you expected, and how long did it take for you to complete one minute?

_____

_____

_____

_____

_____

Day 2

Did you find that your mind kept bouncing all over before you realized it was happening?

_____

Did any particular thought keep taking over? If so, what was it?

_____

How many times did you have to start over?_____

Describe your second attempt here. Was it harder or easier than you expected? Did you get frustrated? How long did it take?

_____

_____

_____

_____

Did you find that during the day, you reminded yourself to focus on the moment or practice the listening?_____
If not yet, you will. You are one day closer to smiling every day.

Day 3

Did you find that your mind kept bouncing all over before you realized it was happening? _____
Did any particular thought keep taking over? If so, what was it?

_____

How many times did you have to start over?_____
Describe your third attempt here: Was it harder or easier than you expected? Did you get frustrated? How long did it take?

_____

_____

_____

_____

Did you find that during the day, you reminded yourself to focus on the moment or practice the listening?_____

Day 4

Did you find that your mind kept bouncing all over before you realized it was happening?_____
Did any particular thought keep taking over? If so, was it a problem or a recurring dialogue with another person?

_____

How many times did you have to start over?_____
Describe your fourth attempt here: Was it harder or easier than you expected? Did you get frustrated? How long did it take?

_____

_____

_____

_____

Did you find that during the day, you reminded yourself to focus on the moment or practice the listening?_____

Day 5

Was your mind bouncing all over before you realized time passed? _____
Did any particular thought keep taking over? If so, what was it?

_____

How many times did you have to start over?_____
Describe your fifth attempt here: Was it harder or easier than you expected, did you get frustrated, how long did it take?

_____

_____

_____

_____

Did you find that during the day, you reminded yourself to focus on the moment or practice the listening?_____

Will you commit to practicing for one to five minutes each morning? If so, be sure to brag about it on my "10 Seconds to Happy" Facebook page. You deserve it. And I will enjoy hearing about your progress.

If you don't feel ready, or if disturbing memories/thoughts came up during your practice, cut yourself some slack; that is not uncommon. Just practice deep breathing and relaxing for fifteen seconds throughout your day until you can progress longer. This is just the beginning of a wonderful ongoing journey, not a task to be completed. If you have any reservations about attempting meditation/mindfulness, search the Internet about it or e-mail your questions to me.

CHAPTER

Time to Start *Feeling* Better

ONE MORNING YOUR ALARM CLOCK GOES OFF AS YOU ARE IN THE MIDDLE OF THE MOST AMAZING, WONDERFUL DREAM. You open your eyes and are saddened to discover that whatever you were dreaming is not real. It might be that you were rich or could fly or that a loved one was still alive. Somehow the happiness you can feel in dreams seems more euphoric than anything we can experience on earth. True bliss. I like to believe dreams like that give us a taste of what heaven will be like. In these dreams, our ancient brain is taking over where our thinking brain is silent. No doubting, questioning, or judging in these types of dreams.

Can you fathom how amazing it would be to tap into that kind of power when you are conscious? What would your life be like? All it takes is steering your imagination, Normally, when anything positive happens, your brain simply notices it; it is just a blip on your awareness radar. Typically, dopamine, oxytocin, and serotonin are reserved for bigger experiences such as a raise, a new car, a new relationship, or being on vacation—and of course, those magnificent dreams where there seem to be no boundaries to the high your brain can create.

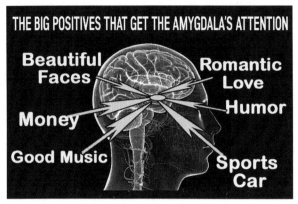

THE BIG POSITIVES THAT GET THE AMYGDALA'S ATTENTION

Beautiful Faces

Romantic Love

Humor

Money

Good Music

Sports Car

As you reset your mind's focus from all that is problematic to all that is good around you, your brain will start to be aware of every positive experience, without you even having to stop and trigger its attention. When I first began my own training, I was blown away when I saw my mind taking charge of finding good around me. Instead of me getting annoyed if something went wrong, my mind instantly would call up all the good around me before I could feel upset. When I first experienced this, I was actually stunned. I stopped in my tracks. "Oh my gosh, it's really happening. *My brain wants to be happy!*" I felt as though someone had taken a warm blanket out of the dryer and wrapped it around me. For the first time, the feeling of peace wasn't fleeting or mysterious. I realized I had just tapped into something life transforming, and I was empowered. It finally clicked that I didn't need to win the lottery to be happy, and I no longer had to fight with all my might to fix whatever was broken. Life would take care of itself if I took care of me.

It took only a couple of months to finally feel what I had been striving for most of my life! *Freedom from the powerful invisible force of emotional fluctuation.* Since that time, I go to sleep with a smile on my face, and I even smile when something goes wrong (most days) because my normal angry emotion isn't anywhere to be found. What I found wasn't just happiness; it was freedom in the truest sense of the word. In the words of dear ol' Janis, "Freedom is just another word for nothing left to lose."—Janis Joplin. I felt no more fear of something happening that would rob me of the things I loved and the peace of mind I so cherished.

This is not positive self-talk; it is different from what you have read in most self-help books and is different from therapy or medication. As I explained in chapter one, thoughts by themselves are no match for feelings that are under the control of adrenaline and cortisol. That is the equivalent of demanding someone who is drunk to *"Sober up right this minute!"*

Those other programs can help you identify your limiting beliefs and biased perspectives, giving you insight, but unless that insight is transferred into emotions, just having an understanding will not yield permanent results.

Most of us have read that book or been at that seminar that really made an impact; however, we had trouble maintaining any real change—often because we had no idea how to keep that powerfully touching information alive or that we should. We often think that just having an epiphany is good enough because the brain will do the right thing with that new information. However, our brains need repeated experiences to create a neural tract that remains.

Although you are reading this book, no matter how many new ideas resonate with you, if you do not practice them each day for at least the first month, they will not rewire your brain. "Repetition is the branding iron of knowledge"as David Toma used to say and that translates into new behavior; your brain already does this to memorize pain and problems from your past, present, and hypothetical future. Now you are going to throw all of that into *REVERSE*.

What Really Makes Humans Happy

Most of us are very confused about what actually makes us happy, which is obvious by our pursuits for the empty promises of status, money, and fame. *In an article published in Harvard Business Review Press in 2011, Professor Amabile states, "We found that of all the events that could make for a great day at work, the most important was making progress on meaningful work — even a small step forward."*

Studies reveal the 3 top things that make humans happy

1. Being a part of something that offers a sense of meaning and purpose. (dopamine/serotonin)
2. Spending time with family and friends. (serotonin/oxytocin)
3. Being kind and helping others. (serotonin/oxytocin)

In short, we need to feel that *we matter*, but when we question our value or those around us do, we can spiral into misery. It doesn't take anything horrible to happen; just having a coworker or supervisor question our competency or having friends go out without inviting us can result in us feeling the darkness creep in. When something like that happens to you, your amygdala trips the switch, telling you death is once again at your doorstep. At that point, you have a few options; as we have discussed, you might create an unrealistic story around what happened to validate your hurt, or you can evaluate the situation against facts until you come to a realistic conclusion that will calm down the cortisol.

The Power of Your Imagination

These investments of your time and energy will be beneficial both in the present and later on, thanks to the amazing power of your imagination. This concept is based on a key insight from neuroscience, that your brain can experience events with the same emotion whether they happen in reality or only in your mind. So, just as you feel bad about past experiences, you can feel good about all of your good experiences by remembering them with full emotion and details. The process and practice of revisiting great experiences with all their details several times a day will establish them as pillars of joy that you can go to whenever you need a break. This focus will also teach your brain that these experiences—not the negative ones—are of utmost importance for your well-being.

How Your Brain Learns to Focus on What You Want

It might seem a bit heady to be retraining your brain's focus on a conscious and subconscious level. However, this happens quite naturally. Have you ever wanted to purchase an item such as a particular car and then suddenly began to see that car everywhere? This happens because you activated your reticular activating system, which seeks and finds whatever you begin to focus on.

You can feel the power of your imagination when you hear your favorite song from high school or encounter an old smell. For me, watermelon lip balm takes me back to the sixth grade and a summer filled with boys and new crushes. How your brain ushers in old memories with all their colors when you hear an old song or encounter a certain smell shows you how powerful imagination is.

Music can transcend present pain, problems, and fear. It sends a signal to the brain that things are going to be OK by releasing dopamine and serotonin. You play a conscious role that cannot be overlooked; when you enjoy a song you love you are giving yourself permission to feel and enjoy the song. Using good/strong memories will be an integral tool in this process. First you need to have and notice great experiences happening to you. Then use the practice of recalling them to reintroduce those same wonderful feelings again, embedding the memory in your brain. As you will see with the music test that follows, memories can be just as powerful as when they first happened.

Let's explore your vacation mind-set. Picture your vacation mind-set as your watermark, the mood you want to recreate and maintain. Yes, it's lofty, but it's doable. If you are like most people, you have tried to keep that calm, chill attitude, promising yourself not to let things get to you anymore when you get back home. It's as though a vacation helps you to see clearly how being stressed has not helped you to be more organized, on time, a better employee, or a better parent. A vacation is the one event that you can count on to calm down the over reactive amygdala. Can you relate to the amazing calm you feel while on vacation even when things go wrong?

My whole family tolerates each other better when we are away. This overriding mind-set of peace and calm is due in part to the *permission* we give ourselves to not care about our schedules or worry about every facet of the day. We let go of expectations, and that decision turns down the alarm bells!

While you are on vacation, you are relaxed; you address any problems that come up and then move on. That pivotal moment when you sit on the beach looking at the waves or the sun or when you ski down that hill with the wind in your hair reaffirms that you do not have to worry at that moment, regardless of the problems facing your life. It's an **official time-out**. Being on vacation is also a validation that you have worked hard and deserve the time-out; it makes you feel **valued**, which is all it takes for serotonin to make you feel **amazing**.

This isn't hard or complicated. We are harnessing the power of your brain by triggering the same brain chemicals that were present during the greatest events of your life.

Your Beliefs, Your Reality

Your beliefs **allow** or **disallow** your wonderful brain chemicals to flow. If you went on vacation but kept telling yourself you didn't deserve it, that you didn't work enough for it, or that you have no money to be on vacation, you would not enjoy yourself. Your belief would supersede the experience, and your brain would not reward you with serotonin. So it is very important that you know what beliefs are active both on the surface and in the background.

Key Beliefs When on Vacation:	
I deserve a time-out.	My only job is to appreciate beauty.
My life won't fall apart.	I can stop worrying.
I need this for my health.	I am safe here.

All of these beliefs can be adopted in everyday life, but until now we have believed that mindset to be opposed to fixing everything we don't like about life.

We are quick to give in to the everyday pressures along with the lie that *we can be happy after these problems are resolved*. Which really just means we will be stressed out until we are back on vacation next year.

To use prior great experiences such as vacations, you simply tap into that wonderful creative mind of yours and remind your brain what vacation feels like, with all the bells and whistles. As you soak in that calm, relaxing, safe feeling, you will be drenching your brain in serotonin and creating a sanctuary you can retreat to when you are dealing with a stressful situation. The rule is that what fires together will wire together. **So as your brain gets accustomed to recalling good experiences when a problem or annoyance arises, it learns very quickly to trigger the release of your happy brain chemicals in the face of stress.** After you have envisioned a bright, detailed memory of your favorite vacation place four or five times a day for at least ten seconds each, it will be a solid memory to pull up when an annoyance arises. That's right, a memory has the power to muffle the warning bells, as you will learn in the next chapter.

Let's Do a Test

Let's see how you can explore these wonderful feelings by triggering them via a song. Get your IPod or whatever you use to listen to music, and find your favorite song. Use a song you have not heard in a while. Sit someplace comfortable. Don't do anything except watch what your brain does...close your eyes, relax, turn it on, and listen. When it ends, continue reading.

Did you feel that? That was your *get happy permission slip!*
Did you notice that you felt a rush of dopamine even at hearing the first few notes? They told you something good was coming—the rest of the song and the memories attached to it. Your brain did not care or differentiate that these were just memories and not happening in the present.

Exercises to Target the Three Areas That Make Us Happy

List organizations in which you could invest your time to help out.

_____

_____

Who are some family and friends you really enjoy and could have on speed dial to spend more quality time with?

_____

_____

What kind of anonymous kind deeds could you do for others?

_____

_____

_____

What projects could you work on that will leave you feeling productive?

_____

_____

Describe a moment you had on vacation when nothing seemed to bother you.

_____

_____

_____

_____

Recall a time while on vacation when things went wrong, but you handled them with grace and patience. Describe how your thinking was different than usual.

_____

_____

_____

_____

Have you ever said to yourself while on vacation, "When I get home and go back to work, I am going to stay calm like I am now and not let things get to me anymore"?

_____

How long was it before you went back to your old reactions? _____
What did it feel like when you realized that your best efforts were thwarted by problems and pressures?

_____

_____

_____

_____

Lets Brighten Up That Vacation Memory

Take a moment now to see your favorite vacation spot. Picture it as you are arriving. Feel the excitement of being off duty for the next several days. Smell the air, hear the sounds, see the other people relaxing, see all the beauty, the scenery and the things unique to that place. Do this for two to three minutes until you are smiling or feeling a warm, calming sensation in your body. A smile tells you it's working. Can you see how quickly your brain responds to a mere memory? Sit with it now and take a time-out. It's OK to feel like you are there right now. If you do it right, you will not be disappointed when you reopen your eyes; don't worry. No need to explain this to anyone, either. This is your safe place. You always tell yourself that you should have a vacation once a month anyway, so take one now. On the next page, write out every detail. The more details you have, the stronger it will be. If you need to write it out before imagining it, do that.

_____

_____

_____

The Best Things in Life Are Free

What stops you from feeling the things you already have? You have worked hard for your home, car, job, friends, and family. When you were growing up, all you could do was dream about one day having these things. Now these things are available to you plus a host of other nice things, good things, great things, and kind things—but as I said earlier, your mind barely notices them. Your brain has been programed to want to just move on so you can get to the next thing. It never ends; its appetite for the **next thing** is insatiable. It sees almost everything as a means to an end...some evasive "end" that never comes, like tomorrow. *At best, it will see each moment as a tool; at worst, as another problem to be solved or overcome.*

This is the dreary fog in which we walk around in, never really seeing, feeling, or tasting any of the precious things life brings to us. This has to change. We must understand that the degree to which we give this moment our *full attention* and *focus* will be the degree to which the next moment is prepared for us. Life is not a series of obstacles to get through every day. For what? When does the pleasure start? When we get home from work? When we get the kids to bed? When we get into bed? The pleasure is hiding in plain view within each moment we experience. The pleasure is recognizing that there is no other place to be but *in this moment*. It is the pleasure of not running ahead worrying about stuff that has not even happened, the pleasure of seeing the smiles on the faces of friends and colleagues that we normally only glance at. This pleasure entails smiling right now and knowing things don't have to be perfect to feel good right now. Today we must come out of this fog and never allow it to control our attitudes and moods again.

Let's talk about how to release these wonderful brain chemicals DOS so that you can feel the way you felt on vacation. First, I will cover the kinds of experiences and memories you can start to soak in that will help to release DOS; however, remember that just having positive experiences is not enough. They pass through your brain like an invisible vapor; meanwhile, your brain grabs hold of all the negative stuff as though it were its best friend. You need to engage with each positive experience by pausing to actively weave it into the brain. I will show you how.

Let's start with your current conditions. Look around and see all the good and safe conditions of this present moment (e.g., you are alive, human, and not in a war zone; you have food to eat, and you are warm, dry, cool, and clean with a roof over your head; you can listen to music and are able to drive and walk). The key here is to feel the same amount of positive emotion toward these things as you would experience negatively if they weren't there. Remember, using these good feelings to trigger DOS is the cornerstone of this practice. Just thinking about them, talking about them, or remembering them **will not** work because these brain chemicals, DOS, are not released by your prefrontal cortex, the thinking part of your brain. They are only released by the limbic system, your emotional center, so you have to try to **feel** these good things to trigger their release.

Identify Your Brain's Bias

On a scale of 1-10 notice how much emotion the following situations raise: See how upbeat you feel, with 10 being upbeat" and 1"not at all," This is not about how you see them but how you **feel** them register in your mind.

The Start of Your Day:

Wake up on time	1 2 3 4 5 6 7 8 9 10
Feel rested	1 2 3 4 5 6 7 8 9 10
Had a nice breakfast	1 2 3 4 5 6 7 8 9 10
Kids off to school on time	1 2 3 4 5 6 7 8 9 10
Car started	1 2 3 4 5 6 7 8 9 10
No line at coffee shop	1 2 3 4 5 6 7 8 9 10

Now do the same exercise for the events below. Notice how much emotion the following situations raise: See how upset you feel as you read these.

The Start of Your Day:

Wake up late	1 2 3 4 5 6 7 8 9 10
Feel exhausted	1 2 3 4 5 6 7 8 9 10
Raining hard outside	1 2 3 4 5 6 7 8 9 10
No time for breakfast	1 2 3 4 5 6 7 8 9 10
Kids wake up late, are cranky	1 2 3 4 5 6 7 8 9 10
Car won't start	1 2 3 4 5 6 7 8 9 10
Long line at coffee shop	1 2 3 4 5 6 7 8 9 10

Do you see how much higher your numbers are toward the negative outcomes? Can you see how your brain is programmed to respond more to problems than to the good things?

For every experience that elicits a negative emotion at six or above, your goal is to be that happy about those events when they go <u>right</u> every day.

It is important to note that the reason we need more than just a few examples to practice every day is one; dopamine effects like the others are short lived, and two; dopamine is triggered when something is new or novel. Once it is commonplace, your brain will not respond the way it did the first time—but that is fine because every day there are plenty of new good things to find. The fact that you will be on the lookout for them will prepare your brain to be in the ready position. Your brain likes habits. That is why they are so hard to break. So being in this habit of seeing the good things around you, fresh and with appreciation, is what will train your brain to have this new positive outlook.

Stop the Hurry and Worry

Taking the time to absorb all the good around you will cause you to physically slow down, in a good way. You will be less hurried and calmer. You need be aware whenever you begin to start rushing around in a hurried fashion. When that happens, you are not appreciating the positive and have gone on autopilot. Remember, physically moving too quickly, hurrying about the office or kitchen, or driving too fast means you are not present, and are rushing toward some future event.

After a few weeks of practicing mindfulness/meditation, you will notice that when you are done, you feel calmer and have greater awareness. As you continue practicing, you will end the session having a more peaceful state of mind. You will find your thoughts no longer racing along but rather absorbed in the present, freeing you to pay attention to what you are doing. At first, it will fascinate you that your thoughts are not sweeping you away. Instead, your mind will seem completely interested in what you are doing in the moment. Regardless of what that is, you will find a contentment in just being with it.

The moment this happens, you will have an "aha" moment: "This is what it feels like to have my mind under my control." Now don't be dismayed; this peace of mind will slip away and your brain will initially resort back to its old patterns, but over time the peace of mind will last longer and longer.

I remember rushing around one morning trying to get out of the house. I was trying to remember what I had to take with me when I realized I had forgotten to empty the dishwasher. I stopped dead in my tracks and felt the aggravation start, but as I opened up the dishwasher and saw the clean glasses and dishes, my brain—now being on the lookout for anything good—paused. I had a choice at that point whether to say, "Never mind this; I need to get out of here!" Or remind myself that my happiness is all I care about since it is the reason I do everything to begin with. I chose the latter. I took a deep breath and allowed myself to feel how good it was to have a working dishwasher. I then took a moment to feel how annoying it would be to have a sink full of dirty dishes and no way to quickly clean them. I took another breath and handled each piece with care and appreciated the use of each, imagining how it would be if I had no glasses or dishes to begin with. My brain at this slower, investigative pace seemed completely absorbed in how each piece looked, felt, and was designed. In only seconds I didn't care that I might be a few minutes late because I was feeling happy, safe, secure, and (most important) in control of my own emotions. That was the perfect way to start my day.

Your job is to **STOP** rushing past these good experiences. I find that when I am out running errands, rushing can get the best of me. Back when I was first learning all of this, I was at the grocery store and needed one item but had to wait in a long line. As I felt indignation welling up with all of my judgments, I just stopped. I reminded myself that the trail my mind was about to go down would in *no way* make me feel good, and because I had committed to focusing only on thoughts that make me feel good, I owed it to myself to just stop. I felt the bottom of my feet on the floor. Pushing all my attention there calmed me down quickly. I then had a wonderful feeling of strength and confidence as I realized I was growing more and more in control of my reactions.

The Modern Marvels We Take for Granted

Let me put into perspective the absurdity of our tendency to quickly dismiss our modern-day advancements. We complain when it takes an extra twenty seconds to send an e-mail. Twenty seconds to send our thoughts, which may or may not be of any importance to anyone but us, to the other side of the world! When I was growing up, it blew my mind to hear another voice on the other end of my new walkie-talkies that I got for Christmas. What about Facebook's occasional changes? OMG, everyone starts flipping out as if it will stop the world as we know it, and the "I am leaving Facebook forever" chant begins. This program allows us to find in mere minutes a second grade crush! And for free! Our storming off is pretty much irrelevant to Facebook, yet our overinflated perception of our own influence is staggering!

How about an IPad? I admit I have flipped out when it takes too long to get on YouTube. I've gotten indignant at how it is interrupting my workout on the stationary bike because I have no use for the twelve TV channels that the gym offers. It is all because I want what I want when I want it. And what I want is to be watching lectures from UCLA while I exercise!

When you take a moment to think about how you have reacted over these stupid little interruptions, you have to either laugh or feel kind a dumb. Your choice.

Starting today, make sure a positive experience or modern marvel is never wasted again. Right now, look around and notice five things that are there for you in any way. These are your good facts. They may be from the past, present, or future. They could be people, surroundings, or technology. Perhaps one thing is your cell phone that lets you see the other person's face while you talk to them. Bluetooth technology that allows you to answer your phone through your car speakers. Your computer—do I even need to say anything about that? What about a GPS that can keep you from getting lost even if you are 3,000 miles from home?

Then there is all the various social media and how it keeps you in touch with everyone and everything that matter to you and on a screen that fits into your pocket! There are also all of the things you are able to accomplish each day because of technology. Things you do with ease that make your day run smoothly or allow you make a living.

I never stop being amazed that I can ask any question on the Internet that I think of and can get multiple answers, in less than a second! I remember my days at the town library and how lucky I was if they had the book I was looking for; usually I was told they had to rent it from some other library six towns away. Now I can find the answer to things I would never dare even ask in public!

The Power of a Compliment

We are quick to overestimate the size of our problems and to underestimate our resources for handling them. We also downplay the good things done for us and to us, such as compliments or kind gestures. Just as we learn to be aware of the small things that trigger bad moods, we must be aware of those things that could trigger a good mood.

Years ago, it was brought to my attention that I often ignored nice things being said to me. When I began to see this, I couldn't believe how much I blew them off.

Compliments are just one small thing that can make a very subtle change in your mood. Instead of discounting things like compliments, you are going to build a habit of replaying them, letting them really sink in. This will begin to increase your self-confidence. In addition, you might notice the other person's countenance lift. People like to have their compliments received, but many of us have not learned how to handle compliments gracefully. We are quick to downplay the nice things people say to us, and we sometimes even make disparaging remarks about ourselves, especially about our looks. This really makes the other person feel disconnected from us.

I once realized that many of the great things I noticed about people I never actually said to them. To break this habit of keeping nice thoughts to myself, I got in the habit of calling or emailing people after I got home to tell them whatever I noticed. It made their day every time.

The Little Things

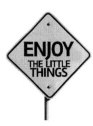

Look for items in your immediate surroundings that are relaxing, comforting, inspiring, informative, or helpful. Look at your outdoor surroundings and the beautiful trees or warm faces that you see. If outdoors is not an option, see if you can see or feel something beautiful, like a picture on the wall, a comfortable chair, or even the sturdy floor. Think of something or someone you are glad to have apart of your life in your present or past. Think of how easy it is to find decent, clean clothes. What would it be like if you had to walk a mile right now in order to get water from a well. Ponder for just a moment the images you see on TV of homeless, sick, hungry, and hopeless people. Focusing for the first time with real attention on any of these things I just mentioned will change your mood in just moments. Once I went over to a neighbors house across the street. I almost never go over there. I stood on their porch and looked over at my house. I couldn't believe how nice it really looked. It was like I was seeing it for the first time. Do the same with your own home.

Over the next few weeks, this constant awareness of good things as well as the choice to keep small setbacks in perspective will simply begin to increase the presence of DOS. You will feel less afraid of "the other shoe dropping," you will stop yourself before you worry about events in the future, and you will feel less uptight because you have a way to handle problems better than ever before. **Your brain will not overreact because you have been forcing it to take notice of so much good around you that your good brain chemicals will be taking precedence, maintaining a state of gratitude and peace.**

How Your Mind Will Argue

Habits and neural patterns die hard and your inner drama queen always wants to assess what is more important by determining the threat level. So your efforts to focus on warm, fuzzy facts might be met with two simple words: "So what." The debate might go something like this: "You have clean sheets; so what? You still have no money to pay your electric bill." Or "So what, you still don't know what the test results will be." Or "So what, you still need to find a new car."

Remember, you are not trying to fix those situations at this time. Your only goal is to ward off the emotional effects of the adrenaline and cortisol triggered by your amygdala, by filling your synapses with DOS instead. Don't fall into the mental trap of weighing the importance of a good feeling against a current problem. It will always feel that the problem should take precedence, but that is irrelevant. Your job is to feel safe and secure and focus only on facts so that you stop speculating on disaster. You are not ignoring the issues you are facing; you are simply soaking your brain in the good stuff, like anesthetic, so that you can feel better. And if you tell me you are worried that you will become a nitwit smiling all day on a park bench, that is like telling me you don't want to join a gym because you don't want to look like a bodybuilder!

Appreciation Exercise:

See how upset you would be if the things listed below happened. Read the list below and pause at each one to imagine experiencing each event, with all the details and emotions you would feel. Imagine how crummy it would be to have to deal with them and how they would affect your day (Take time for this; it's important.)

Rip in Your Pants	Big Stain on Couch
Lost Wallet	Dent on Car
Lost Keys	Earrings are Missing
Spilled Coffee in Car	Car Won't Start
Cell Phone Missing	Virus That Wipes Computer Out

Now take ten to fifteen seconds with each one to imagine each problem disappearing, allowing yourself to feel relieved. Let it really sink in how really wonderful it is that these situations are not something you have to deal with today.

Every day, their absence and the absence of other things like them are a GOOD experience, a blessing that you need to soak in. Try to even name the good feelings you experience (e.g., wonderful, safe, secure, appreciative, happy). Allowing these feelings of appreciation and gladness to soak in will begin to reset your brain's spotlight so it gets in the habit of looking for the good things all around you rather than letting them simply go unnoticed.

Practice Being in The NOW Right Now

1. Pay attention to every positive fact around you. Register each thing deeply in your mind's attention by saying it out loud: "I feel safe in this chair. I am protected by these walls. I feel the warm clean air that I'm breathing." Write each fact down.

_____

_____

_____

_____

_____

_____

_____

_____

_____

2. Now pick another fact. For example, I have family who love me, friends who care, kids, or something similar. Now close your eyes for ten seconds and savor it. Feel it emotionally to intensify it, just as you would do in your mind if you were angry. Don't rush. Ten seconds is just a guideline; go for twenty if you can. In the early stages, taking a longer time to feel the sensation will train the brain faster.

3. Feel it soaking into your brain and body, registering it deeply as an emotional memory. When you smile or feel as though there is a warm blanket around you, you've nailed it. If you want to speed up the rewiring process, do this at least twice

an hour for one minute. In the beginning you will have to remind yourself to do it, but after just one week, it will become natural and you will be doing it several times per hour, feeling more and more appreciative and fortunate. *Make up your mind to practice, and your brain will do the rest.*

In the words of Abraham Lincoln, *"Most folks are about as happy as they make their minds up to be"*. So make up your mind now!

Time To Soak it In

Bring to mind a person who cares for you, loves you, and genuinely wishes you well. Feel the person's love and concern for you. Bring to mind anything that makes you feel peaceful, relaxed, happy, or loved, or think of a pet or child you love. Now take ten seconds or more for each thing you noticed, feeling their goodness sinking into you. Wait for that smile. When you are done, write them out below. Comment on anything you never noticed before.

1 _____

_____

2 _____

_____

3 _____

_____

4 _____

_____

5 _____

_____

Here are some great things that we take for granted. Each morning find three things around you to focus on and feel good about—or use the list below—before you leave the house. It will help if you preface each event or item that you use with the thought of how it would feel to **not** have these things.

Morning:

- Appreciate a pair of socks that you like and the fact that they are clean without holes.
- If it is a nice day, appreciate the warmth of the sun and clean air.
- If it is rainy or snowy, appreciate that you have a warm house or a dry car to get you around safely.
- Appreciate having food for breakfast or the money to buy a cup of coffee.
- Even if your morning is hectic getting the kids out the door, appreciate that they are healthy and can get to school without physical assistance. Some parents will never know what that is like, and considering that for just a minute or two will calm your nerves when your kids are dragging their feet.
- If you are a parent with a disabled child, know that this child will teach you more about ways to smile than a hundred books could.
- Notice and feel good about having enough makeup, soap, even deodorant. Running out of any of those things during your morning routine would be a real pain, so be sure to appreciate every moment those things come together for you.
- Appreciate having clean clothes regardless of whether they are exactly what you like to wear.

Afternoon:

- Feel good when things ARE NOT damaged or broken. Initially this will feel unimportant. This is where you will be rewiring things.

- Feel good when your car starts right up.

- Really enjoy driving to work and having no traffic jams. You know how furious you can become when there is traffic, so take note when there is none.

- Smile with pleasure and appreciation when your computer starts up and behaves.

- Got a ton of e-mails to go through? Take a moment to revel in the amazing technology that lets you send a message to a person three cubicles down faster than you can walk there.

- For women, a bad hair day can really put us in a mood, so girls, when you're having a good hair day, remind yourself several times a day how wonderful your hair looks.

- Take time for lunch, reminding yourself that you deserve to eat and take a break. Focus on the taste, texture, and nutrition.

- If you had an anxiety-producing morning and need to calm down, find a local pet store at lunch and ask if you can play with a puppy or kitten. Think about nothing but giving the pet some love and your oxytocin will explode, which is the best thing for calming stress.

- Feel great about getting a close parking space; don't rush past it but rather sit there for a few seconds and let it sink in.

- Be present and really enjoy a great conversation with a loved one.

- Be thankful for finding some extra money in a wallet or pocket.

- Soak in having had a hard laugh with a friend or coworker.

- Notice how you feel after buying yourself a luxury item. Really memorize how that feels. Shopping kicks in dopamine, which is why people get addicted to it…OK, women get addicted.

- Be thankful when you purchase the last item on the shelf.

- For women, when you get that manicure, truly enjoy it, let it sink in, and admire how pretty your nails look. We spend a fortune and then appreciate them for only an hour or so.

- Sitting down to dinner is not something you should rush through, thinking only about getting the kitchen clean and watching TV.
- Be thankful that you have the ingredients to make the meal you just decided to make.
- Pay attention to the conversation at dinner as though you never heard those voices before. (It helps to pretend you are in a dream)
- Be thankful that the kids are healthy and tucked in.
- Be happy that the house is secured and locked.
- Be thankful that you are fed, not hungry.
- Appreciate that you had clean water to take a relaxing shower.
- At night, take it in when climbing into a bed with clean sheets and putting on clean pajamas.

Again, savor these by taking in every detail of them, and visit the opposing options to feel the reality of their goodness.

This is the whole crux of rewiring your brain and mind. With this reserve of DOS in your synapses, you will handle problems with a vacation mind-set.

End-of-Day Journal:

Each night before bed, look back over your day and write things down, starting with the evening and working backward. Recount all the good things that you may have missed. Then ask yourself if anything happened that motivated or encouraged you about your life or even mankind. Did anything good happen that you did not expect? Did you see, feel, or hear anything that pulled at your heartstrings that maybe you overlooked? Do this every night for one month, and it will change your life. You can write your first night out here. (By the way this one practice alone has been proven in studies to lift the mood of even clinically depressed people.)

_____

_____

_____

_____

_____

_____

End of Week Journal:

Look back over the past week and ask yourself how many issues you worried about or got upset over that never manifested. See if you can remember five things you overstressed about that worked out better than you initially expected. Even if it was something as small as being late somewhere, your car making a funny noise, or being worried that someone might be mad at you.

If you have any trouble remembering things, perhaps that is because they worked themselves out or never materialized, and instead of your brain reminding you to feel good about them, it simply dismissed them and moved on to the next thing to worry about. This practice will help you catch yourself during the day before you are getting worked up unnecessarily

1 _____

2 _____

3 _____

4 _____

5 _____

A SHORT PICK ME UP LIST

It is good to have some things handy that can increase DOS quickly for those sudden drops in mood. Here are some things you can experience quickly to bring about a dopamine, serotonin, or oxytocin release. Keep them handy for those sudden tough moments.

I remember once in high school I was so sick of the Jersey winter that when I saw our Coppertone suntan lotion on the shelf one morning, I took it down and took a big whiff. Wow. I was transported right to the beach. So I wondered what would happen if I put some around my neck. Well, I did, and for a few days it was amazing; I would just close my eyes and feel like it was a summer day. The really funny part was that when a few of my friends smelled it, half of them teased me, but the others kept sniffing me, saying it made them happy.

- Take a good whiff of your favorite suntan lotion in the middle of a dreary winter day.
- The smell of your favorite lotion, incense, or candle can do wonders. Aromatherapy through essential oil blends with names like "Peace and Calming" or "Valor" that can change your mood when diffused. Any one of these at your desk will do more for you than a piece of candy or carb snack.
- Write your own smell ideas here that you can keep around.
- Chew your favorite kind of gum.
- Hug someone. A twenty-second hug will raise your oxytocin level.
- Name three people you can count on for great hugs.

1 _____

2 _____

3 _____

- Have a great night of sex. Oxytocin seems to be able to alleviate strong anxiety better than dopamine or serotonin.
- The sound of birds chirping can be wonderfully relaxing and is also very helpful to have as a soundtrack playing in your cubicle.
- Download nature sounds to your phone.
- Exercise three times a week with thirty minutes of aerobics, if you are able to. After about a month, you will notice the endorphins keeping you calmer for forty-eight to seventy-two hours. If you hate working out, use music. Like I have said exercise can do more for mood that some anti-depressants.
- Laughter can also kick endorphins in. Take ten to fifteen minutes to watch funny videos from YouTube.
-

List three of your favorite funny videos that you have saved to your watch list on YouTube. Find three if you don't already have them.

1 _____

2 _____

3 _____

Buy a small luxury item for yourself. List six small affordable things you could buy (e.g., lip balm or lip gloss, your favorite cereal, a new lotion, a new book, a rented movie, new shampoo, a magazine, an accessory for the car or tool).

_____

_____

Until now, I have been generalizing about good feelings. However, we need to dive a bit deeper because when we feel an overriding emotion, we need to know what chemical it might be affecting. We have three basic areas of necessity that the brain is always assessing.

Those three areas are:

Dopamine- Food/Water —— Oxytocin- Inclusion/Love- Serotonin/Security

When something happens that throws you off your game, you need to first assess which of the above areas it is affecting and then grab for the exact counter emotion. To experience the positive counter emotion, you need recall counter experiences or engage in certain behaviors. So it helps to have them handy. Review the list below, and then recall your own positive emotions or experiences that would match the description on the right. This is a key technique for bad moments or bad days. Then write down the actual experiences you can remember.

Positive Emotions or Behaviors to Use Against Negative Feelings

Threatened	Safe, secure, guarded
Attacked	Protected
Sad	Grateful
Depressed/hopeless	Need a new perspective. Call or go visit someone to help
Unsatisfied/negative	Complete a task or project. Call or visit someone you can help.
Weak / Helpless	Strong, accomplished
Devalued	Appreciated, Involved

On the following pages write down all of the wonderful ways you experience your needs being met.

Experiences Having Ample Food and Water

_____

_____

_____

_____

_____

_____

_____

_____

_____

_____

_____

_____

_____

_____

_____

_____

_____

_____

_____

_____

Experiences of Having Loving Moments with People or Pets

Experiences of Feeling Safe, Secure, and Protected

_____

_____

_____

_____

_____

_____

_____

_____

_____

_____

_____

_____

_____

_____

_____

_____

_____

_____

_____

_____

EXPERIENCES THAT CAN LOWER YOUR DOPAMINE

Rejection by a potential or existing lover or friends

Laying around the house doing nothing

Loss of food source

Grief and loss of friendship or death of person or pet

Loss of job or money

Team Loss

Car accident

Serious disappointment after buying an expensive item

EXPERIENCES THAT CAN LOWER YOUR OXYTOCIN

Rejection of a lover or close friend

Lack of physical touch

Isolation, being rejected, or having a disagreement

Lack of emotional exchange

Intense stress

Feeling misunderstood or disconnected, having a friend angry with you

Having your last child leave the nest

Having your favorite show cancelled

EXPERIENCES THAT CAN LOWER YOUR SEROTONIN

Being around others who brag

Your boss being unhappy with you

Feeling less smart or good looking, feeling inferior to others

Comparing what you have to what others have (money, possessions, spouse, etc.).

Feeling poor not having the money to buy something in the moment

Feeling left out or excluded

Seeing others win, accomplish, or get ahead

Not getting things accomplished you had planned

Being fearful you overspent

Having someone correct you in public (anything embarrassing)

These are just a few examples that can lower some of your brain chemicals. For years, you may have found that you came home feeling awful after being in certain circumstances or around certain people. Now you can start to figure out what was triggering that feeling by reviewing your three core areas and increase the chemical that seems to be affected prior to being in those situations.

For the Women Readers

Even after practicing these techniques for a few years, during that time of the month, some women can suddenly find that focusing on good things isn't registering. During this time, norepinephrine and epinephrine (also known as adrenaline and noradrenaline) have kicked in, and you may feel tenser, more uptight, and more impatient. Being sure to take the time in the morning and in the afternoon to soak in good things for a longer period will be key. I don't deny that I could be the poster child for PMS misery; I notice the good, but I don't feel it as much. If this happens to you, it is not your fault. Nothing is wrong, but you will have to ride this out for a couple of days. I have also found that when I have soaked my brain in DOS prior to that time, I do much better. (For years I have been recommending to clients to take 1000mg of the amino acid Tyrosine on an empty stomach to calm down norepinephrine and epinephrine. It works like magic in about 2 hours.

10

CORNERSTONE OF HAPPINESS— FINDING *Your* PURPOSE

THE IMPORTANCE OF HAVING A PURPOSE IN LIFE CAN'T BE OVERSTATED, AND FOR GOOD REASON. Like I said in chapter seven scientific studies have proven time and time again that the happiest people in the world are those who feel they have a purpose. We need to matter.

That purpose can involve the world, your town, your family, or any organization where you feel needed or counted on. When that wanes, even in the course of a day, it can leave you experiencing low-grade misery. To the degree that you feel you make a difference, you will feel good. Purpose is why humans are drawn to join clubs, groups, fraternities, sororities, and other organizations.

In the course of your day, the short-term purposes may be obvious; your lifelong purpose, however, can be more obscure. Yet when you know what yours is, it will be the reason you spring out of bed in the morning.

Many people have no idea what their purpose is, and tons of seminars are given every year to help them find it. Not knowing one's purpose can trigger a midlife crisis and can be the reason for taking trips to go find oneself. We all seem to have this innate need to know that there is a reason—and a damn good one—for being on this earth. Often this issue raises its head only long after college, as in college goals have more to do with career choice and making money; much less consideration is given to the importance of making a difference.

I often work with troubled youth. I don't look for them or hang out a shingle, but they seem to find me. They are the special ones, the ones I feel blessed to know. Each is so unique and powerful in his or her own way but derailed for a season by drugs or parents who couldn't even take care of a gerbil. I avail myself 24/7 to these kids, whether to help with dinner, homework, or lunch money, or even to help them find a college. Endless hours of therapy/discussion transpire to help them move on into the next phase of their life. Everyone of them learn quickly that there is a reason they are alive; a mandate to fill that no one else can. When this truth clicks for them they become empowered and confident ready to try anything. This foundation will also keep them from getting derailed years later by chasing some elusive material possession or status.

The twofold blessing is that in teaching them these values, I also gain a sense of purpose for myself. However, with all of that, I can still have a week of feeling as though I am not making a difference. Those days and weeks are uncomfortable but certainly not accurate. Even a lifelong purpose can lose its luster and its feel-good qualities if we don't feel we are making a tangible difference we can feel at that moment. We need that validation that recharges our batteries and says, "You absolutely make a difference." I know we are adults and should be able to keep our own motivating fire stoked, but we need it from our "tribe" as well.

It feels amazing when your superior pulls you aside or better yet, overhearing someone say what a difference you make for them.

The way to persevere and break through the moments when you are questioning your worth is to find something to do that will give you a sense of purpose in the moment. Believe it or not, all that may be required is that you clean out the garage. You might think that pales in comparison to a "change the world" kind of purpose, but remember, your brain doesn't care what exactly you accomplish. It just likes for you to accomplish things it can see and feel. Ask any cleaning nut, and he will confirm that he loves to see the difference his efforts make. When I was a kid, every Saturday my sister and I had chores. I always wanted to do the vacuuming, and she was fine with that. One day she asked, "That is harder; why do you like it?" I said, "Because I can see the difference the vacuum makes."

When people can't find their purpose, they may seek relief by drinking, smoking pot, being promiscuous, or having an affair—as so many Hollywood stars have exemplified. After this, clinical symptoms may even appear, such as outright depression, anxiety, and even self-harm.

What It Feels Like to Lose Your Purpose

Without purpose and direction, you can start to flounder and experience feeling bored, restless, or blah, with little satisfaction. Feelings of guilt may surface, but you will not be sure why. You will want to go back to bed. You might feel unloved, unnoticed, unlovable. You might even feel disgusted, hating your life and yourself. Nothing underscores how bad this can feel as people who feel so little purpose that they commit suicide. And nothing underscores how misguided their feelings and thoughts can be as in the death of Robin Williams. The whole world could have told him he mattered but due to a chemical imbalance he had no way to feel it or verify it. Never trust your feelings, always check your facts. Everyone matters!

Losing a sense of your life's purpose and desperately trying to find one can place you in a revolving paradoxical mind-set...one minute believing you could accomplish anything, given the chance, and the next minute feeling that you have very little to offer the world. It is within this dichotomy that a miserable life evolves. I don't personally know anyone who does not succumb to this at one time or another swinging between these two paradigms sometimes in the course of a day. You may be unaware of this trigger and attribute your low-grade mood to being tired, bad weather, problems, or stress at home and work. By learning to stay aware of what is going on in your head, with mindfulness you will be able to ascertain what erroneous thoughts are floating around and address them quickly. Then you can find or create a purpose in the moment and be rewarded with a nice shot of self-esteem and well-being, thanks to serotonin. In fact, the sense of accomplishment is so tied to a good mood that often if you are in a bad mood, just deciding to accomplish some kind of task can snap you out of it.

If you have been feeling like you have no purpose but have been searching, I applaud you. This is not a journey for the faint of heart. It takes fearless exploration, with no excuses. Writing down your goals for the month and staying aware of them throughout is a key step.

Whenever I am starting to flounder for more than a month, I usually find that I lost my direction because I lost sight of my goals. When I need to fix this, I spend a whole Sunday writing out pages of ideas, dreams, goals, and accomplishments that I still want to pursue, and in the middle of all these, my message and purpose will resurface. A specific purpose may unfold and define itself over the course of a month or a year, but that is where it starts for me. Everything I have written will light my path whenever I get cloudy on direction or feel that I am not doing enough with my life.

Moment to Moment Purpose

Every time a group of scientists does a study to find the happiest employees in the world, the answer is always the same: those whose responsibilities impact their colleagues the most. The ones who troubleshoot and figure out the problems of others report having the most pleasure in their lives and jobs.

Being the hero for a few moments, the feeling of being needed, provides you with a sense of accomplishment, via the neurotransmitter serotonin. Any opportunity to influence another person or your environment will make you feel, secure, confident, and proud, lifting your spirits in a matter of seconds.

For various reasons, we can all find ourselves sinking during the day. A common mistake we all make is to personalize these blah moods, as in, "Uh oh, something must be wrong, something I don't know about yet." I used to take a nap when these moods hit, and that often helped, but now I know I can impact it directly. *It's never personal; it's simply chemical.*

Don't psychoanalyze these passing moods, looking for some big, hidden issue. Most days it is just a chemical that you need to fire up. Evolution has proven over time that humans survive only by helping each other, so a strong drive evolved within us that leads us to try to make things better, support, collaborate, and make a difference for an optimum life.

Simply look around for anyone who might need your wisdom, sense of humor, love, hug, encouraging word, or physical assistance. Call a friend whom you know could use an ear, some wisdom, or a laugh. Not just any friend; it has to be someone struggling. If no one comes to mind, go on Facebook and search through your friends to find someone struggling. Send the person a private message or give them a call; if you lift their mood in any way, I guarantee you will feel more valued and enriched, relieving that sense of no-purpose.

In a famous research study, people were given $20 and then asked to give that same $20 away while they were hooked up to electrodes. What the study revealed was that the brain's reward center lights up with more activity when people give someone else $20 than when they receive it! It truly is better to give than to receive!

Doing a good deed or showing a perfect stranger some kindness will make you feel better, regardless of your own situation not changing. You can help carry stuff to someone's car or ask a neighbor if he needs something from the store. This is how AA got started, one alcoholic helping another, and is why it is still so successful today. At an AA meeting, you can find people feeling stronger and lowering their overwhelming urge to drink simply by reaching out to help someone else. AA is a serotonin and oxytocin haven.

Find your story, and you will find your purpose. You have lived a life like no other. Whether boring, exciting, trivial, or grand, your experiences give rise to the same emotions and questions we all strive to answer. Your message is not in the events but in how you respond to them.

The popularity in becoming a life coach is due in part to millions of people trying to find their purpose. It's coaches finding their purpose, in helping you find yours.

Judy Carter has made her purpose in life (aside from making people laugh) to help people find their purpose by finding their message. For each of us our purpose is often hiding within our life's message. Discovering all the things you have learned that others need to know is a very exciting journey. Her book, "The Message of You" will walk you through each step. It is one of the best books on finding your purpose because your purpose is not "out there" it's inside you waiting to be discovered. This is the gold, the stuff we are supposed to pass down to the next generation to help them advance faster and avoid the pitfalls. Every single one of us has a message, one that is meant for a select group of people who, believe it or not, are desperate to hear it. Start to think about what yours is, and you will find more purpose than you ever dreamed of.

What things do you do to help others that make you feel amazing?
List them in priority order. E.g. helping: children, seniors, disabled, teaching, mentoring, etc

1 _____

2 _____

3 _____

3 _____

5 _____

6 _____

Below, list four tasks around the house that you could accomplish when feeling blah. (cleaning, washing, organizing, throwing things out, etc.). Remember, even if you don't think such an activity will satisfy you, it most likely will.

1 _____

2 _____

3 _____

4 _____

*If you want to feel good then
make others feel good*

11

THE "OTHERS" FRIEND OR FOE?

THE WAY WE BEGIN AND END EACH DAY WITH OUR AMYGDALA SCANNING FOR POTENTIAL PROBLEMS IS THE WAY WE ENTER EVERY SOCIAL SETTING. It's why we invented alcohol. Social settings are notoriously hard for many people, and once again we have evolution to thank for that.

Thousands of years ago, meeting new people could mean extreme danger. A new tribe showing up out of nowhere could mean a battle to the death. Very seldom did a new group of people show up just to say, "Wus Up?"

Now here you are thousands of years later, supposedly much more evolved, and yet the moment you walk into a room, that damn amygdala starts scanning for enemies of all kinds. Remember, you are programmed to survive; now, however, instead of your brain looking for people with clubs, it scans for people who might be judging you, giving you a wrong look, or saying something off-color. In this survival mode, you will compare yourself to them, looking for reasons to feel insecure or embarrassed. The smallest infraction will set off major alarm bells! "Boy, they seemed cold. Why do I always have to say hi first? Why are they staring at me?" Is it any wonder we go running for the bar?

Leave the Guard Dog at Home

To learn to be comfortable in social settings, you first have to leave your guard dog at home. You need to retrain your brain to walk into a room and, at first glance, note everything and everyone in the room *for* you, *not* against you.

Start today being mindful when you enter a public setting. Notice, in the background of your mind, the quiet assumption that people are judging you, even at the supermarket. Almost everyone does this. It is why we walk into a store and avoid most eye contact—and is why they, too, assume we don't want anything to do with them. Our way of protecting ourselves is to either ignore the faces in front of us or begin to judge them back.

Once you start to see just how often you avoid eye contact with strangers, you will spot these underlying tendencies. I am still taken back when I am in a store and I hear a kind voice from a stranger or get a kind look. It is there that I instantly feel my defenses come down and am aware of my own negativity churning away in the background. Have you ever noticed that sometimes even when walking into a family event, you feel a slight hesitation until you get that first hug? Then it's like, "Well, at least one person is glad to see me." Even at functions with acquaintances you can have that sense of being ten years old again about to walk by a group of kids you don't know.

In public gatherings of any kind, your subconscious will be hitting the warning bell continuously—the wrong glance from a friend or foe or even someone whispering into an ear thirty feet away will set your amygdala at the "ready" position. You have to pay attention to what is traveling at light speed through your mind—otherwise, trust me, your mood will fluctuate ten times in a minute.

When you begin to take control of the negative background static and go on the offensive to be kind and nice, you will notice your own fears and insecurity dissolve as well as those of the people around you. This is the psychology behind banks and some stores that have people waiting to greet you at the door.

Let me mention here that being socially accepted is a *much* higher priority for women because it is more hardwired into women's brains than into those of men for the reasons I covered earlier. When you change your own comfort capabilities in social settings, you change how you see the whole world, so it is worth the effort!

I remember being at a wedding where the food was absolutely delicious. They had these little different kinds of chocolate truffles. Now I am going to confess that my appetite is deranged at times, and I really have a hard time reeling myself in if the food is really good. So while I was devouring these things, they asked us to go to our assigned tables and stand there.

Well, I see those little heart-shaped vanilla chocolate truffles on the table, and although no one is even sitting yet, I just have to reach over, grab one, and shove it in my mouth. Across from me is a woman I don't know who is looking at me with utter disgust. Now my amygdala is already screaming and has me sweating before I even realize that I actually just shoved a wad of butter into my mouth! I spent the entire night doing everything I could to win that woman back over to my side. I apologized, joked, and made fun of myself, but nothing worked. As far as that woman was concerned, I was out of the tribe, and all I wanted was to be back in. If I had known why this bothered me so much, I would have been able to laugh it off and not let my amygdala wreck my night.

Using Mindfulness in Social Settings

Applying your new awareness in public settings can be a very eye-opening exercise. Take note if you automatically avoid eye contact when in public. See if you do this in some places but not others. Try to get a sense of whether you are feeling vulnerable, insecure, guilty, or just unwanted. I have noticed how people do this when first walking through the door into my gym, but then they loosen up and start making some eye contact after they begin exercising. Maybe it's the common goal they have there; it's like they remind themselves, "It's OK; I am expected to be here." See if you can name what you are feeling at each place you go. Like the doctor's office, store, bank, post office, gym, or theater.

You may notice that at place where you have to wait to be served, that you tend to see the others as obstacles because typically you have to wait for them to get done before you can be taken care of. Initially, we walk into a store and see how much time this will cost us before we even think about a price. On the opposite side, I have actually noticed slight feelings of guilt when I am in line somewhere and another has to wait for me. (But that could just be my Catholic school guilt; let me know if that happens to you.)

As you walk into public places this week with this new 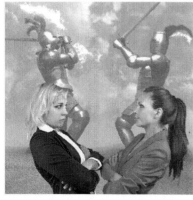 attention, remember that no stranger has any opinion about you, either negative or positive, based in any kind of reality. Most won't even notice you. Observe the people you walk by and how wrapped up in their own world they are. Make eye contact when possible, and smile. When you smile, be prepared to get nothing back but a glare. Do not be dismayed. It is not that common for strangers to be that friendly, especially if you live in the northeast. If you live down south this might be easy for you and quite possibly something you already do. Remember that in some parts of our country people may assume you don't like them, so be mindful of any hidden judgments you may be holding onto.

I know when I smile at someone and am ignored, I have to choose to remember it is not personal. Of course my sarcastic mind wants to say a whole bunch of things, but what I have to protect against the most is the tendency for my subconscious to pull me back from smiling at the next person. I made a decision a long time ago—and sometimes have to remind myself of it five times a day—that I live my life on my terms, not allowing the hurts and beliefs of others to taint my perception.

I want you to make the conscious decision to understand the following: no matter how someone treats you, even if you did something to that person, there are at least a hundred other people who would react differently. People do what they do because of them. It is NEVER about you.

You need to remind yourself of the insecurity and awkwardness many there feel. Do your best to smile with an attitude of letting them know it's safe to be there. See them as the ten-year-old nervous kid meeting new kids for the first time. Watch how fast everyone starts acting warmly toward you as they see that you are approachable and aren't secretly judging them.

I find that specialty stores seem warmest because we feel we have something in common, while food stores are the coldest unless we are buying the same thing.

When I first began to practice walking into stores with a new awareness, I noticed my avoidance with others, and I even realized I had a very subtle attitude toward some actual stores. I live on the east coast, and it is easy to be guarded and skeptical of the agendas of others and even of the store itself. I know it is a business, and I know the owners want to make as much money off me as possible, so my pervasive underlying mood was not one of gratitude. Instead, I felt like I was succumbing to a necessary evil by going there, which made me defensive. I had to change that before I could see the people in the store differently.

Your entire energy field will change for the better and you will know this because complete strangers will begin greeting you with a smile. We are very perceptive creatures and pick up on each others energy faster than you will ever be consciously aware of. As that begins to happen you will gain a new level of confidence in any social setting.

Note: If you have not been doing these exercises, then stop where you are. Just reading this book will do no more than give you "aha" moments, and they don't last. Ask yourself if any hidden beliefs are keeping you from putting in the effort.

On a scale of one to ten (ten being great), how comfortable are you in a social setting before having a drink? **1 2 3 4 5 6 7 8 9 10**

List some of the insecurities, fears, and judgments—real or imagined—that run rampant in your mind. Later, refer back to chapter four and counter them with real facts.

_____

_____

_____

_____

_____

How has this false perception altered your behavior toward people in social settings?

_____

_____

Have you ever judged a person negatively and then discovered he or she was really nice after actually engaging the person in a conversation?

_____

Has anyone ever admitted to you that when they first met you, they really didn't like you but then changed their mind after getting to know you? How did that feel? Did you notice that your own mind is like "What? How could you not like me?"

_____

_____

_____

Think back to a social gathering when you felt overwhelmed and insecure because of your perception and assumptions and not because of an actual event. How did buying into those emotions ruin your time out? What would you do differently now? Explain:

_____

_____

_____

_____

In order to begin this next step you need to get comfortable with the actual physical places that you go into. Start by taking notice of everything there to assist you as soon as you walk into any setting.. At work you might find a comfortable chair, a well-lit desk, a clean bathroom, perhaps some coffee or food. In a store, you might find there are signs to guide you, baskets to help you, proper lighting, or clean shelves. Allow a sense of appreciation to come over you. I mean having to go to a store sure beats having to plunder the woods for something to kill and eat, right? Use the table on the next page to list all the things you noticed that were helpful to you in any way or were simply put there with you in mind. Take ten seconds to let each positive thing you notice soak in until you feel it.

List the place and what you noticed about it.

Venue	Venue	Venue

COMPLETE THIS EXERCISE THROUGHOUT THE WEEK
AS YOU NOTICE YOUR BEHAVIOR.

List the places where you avoid eye contact the most.

_____

_____

Did you avoid eye contact the whole time or only at the beginning? Describe:

_____

_____

Do you avoid eye contact out of any underlying shame or embarrassment, or is it more like a vague insecurity?

_____

_____

In what places do you avoid eye contact the least? Why?

_____

_____

How do you feel when you make eye contact with a stranger?

_____

Does it matter if the stranger is of the opposite sex?

_____

_____

How does it feel when you flash someone a big smile and they smile back as opposed to them looking right through you?

_____

_____

Did any fears rise up as you went to smile at someone?

_____

_____

Describe the first experience in which you noticed other people responding differently toward you.

_____

_____

_____

_____

_____

_____

Did you notice anyone talking to or smiling at you even before you had a chance to smile at them?

_____

_____

_____

Did you have a conversation with anyone with whom you previously wouldn't have engaged in conversation? If so, how did that come about?

_____

_____

_____

Did you notice more of your own judgments? If so, what did you notice first, your negative attitude or the actual thought that preempted it? List them.

_____

_____

_____

_____

Can you recall the specific thought?

_____

_____

12

Turning Lemons Into Lemonade

I AM SURE YOU KNOW NEGATIVE PEOPLE WHO PUT A NEGATIVE SPIN ON EVERYTHING THAT THEY DISCUSS OR RECOLLECT. Even good events can take on a negative tone when recounted by "Downer Dan." Instead of admitting something was good, he somehow finds a way to downplay it. However, there is something to be gleaned from that ingrained pattern. These patterns are learned then perfected by repeated practice and then ingrained. (create neural patterns)

It is that same effort that you will put forth, but in the opposite direction. By putting a spin of gratitude on things (and I don't mean being in denial of bad things happening), your brain will learn very quickly to ingrain that pattern as well. It will begin to review even your memories through your new eyes of gratitude. So when life throws you a curve, instead of your memory trying to recall all the other times things went wrong, it will now recall things that have gone well. Now it is true that some people do this naturally and are just born positive people; they are rare, but I have read about them, so I know they exist.

A while back I was having lunch at a neurobiology conference. The conversation went in the way of discussing car accidents (I guess we needed to dumb it down for lunch), and I mentioned that I was hit by a drunk driver more than fifteen times, also mentioning the physical impairments I was left with. It was a dramatic story of me chasing her for forty minutes until ten cop cars finally caught up and tried to stop us both.

Initially she hit me at over 55 miles per hour while I was stopped at red light. When I got my bearings back, I realized that instead of seeing if I was OK, she was trying to back up her crumpled car so she could get away. Well, thanks to some high quantities of adrenaline and dopamine, I ignored the pain shooting down my back and quickly and could tell she was drunk. I believed that if someone did not stop her, she would likely kill someone. So I decided to help out. As she hit speeds of 80 miles per hour, I pursued her as carefully as I could (no, I really did), but each time I got close enough to see her license plate and tried to call 911, all I got was "still searching" on my phone, Ugh! She repeatedly nodded off at intersections and traffic lights, at which point I would pull my car in front of her and try to block her path, but like a drunk Tasmanian Devil, she would spring to life and slam on the accelerator.

You will have to see me in person to hear the rest of the story, but the point is that at the end of my story, the woman to whom I was telling this looked at me and asked, "Are you angry for what she did to you?" I was caught off guard; no one had ever asked me that before. I said, "Not at all. I feel like that was one of the moments I will look back on as when my life really mattered." That driver had been arrested five times for drunk driving prior to that afternoon. After the accident, she went to prison for a year, got sober, and became a drug counselor. Now she sends me a thank-you card each year on "our anniversary," thanking me for being her guardian angel.

Others at the table commented on my positive attitude. I smiled because until that moment, I had never seen myself as a positive person, persé I always considered myself a realist. It was then that I realized I had always viewed a positive attitude as a decision to forcibly put a positive spin on things. I'd thought it was a decision that took strength and fortitude and a giant fake smile that I always believed was more about being in denial. Conversely, for me in this story, there was no other choice, no pushing away a buried resentment; this was the only way to see it.

As I have now rewired my brain with these techniques, I see that same perception pervading all the areas of my life. Now it just takes pausing for a moment for me to see the reality of all the goodness around me, and there is no other choice but to smile and feel good about life.

After practicing these techniques, your brain, too, will begin to naturally lean toward this perception. It won't take putting rose-colored glasses on—just clear ones.

A Trip Back to the Future

When I was a kid, my friends and I would make up all kinds of games to play. We lived in the country, so we had a lot of freedom to roam around our neighborhood. The most fun we had was when we pretended to be someone else…a rock star, a spy. We played air instruments for hours to the popular songs of the '70s, pretending we were on the Mike Douglas Show, and we rode around on our bikes pretending we were on spy missions.

A rich fantasy life is the treasure of childhood. As girls, it was easy to pretend we were out on a date with Donny Osmond or David Cassidy. I remember how easy it was to get lost in those games for hours and feel satisfied. It was a safe escape from the pressures of fitting in and doing homework. As adults, we realize we have to deal with reality, and we walk away from that precious gift, our imagination.

Well, it's time to use it once again and take a little trip.

After years of feeling that you have been a victim of circumstance, never being given your fair shot at the good life, it can be a challenge to release your grip around the neck of negativity. Even your best efforts can be hindered by stubborn patterns of fear, and it can seem almost impossible to review your life in anything less than the dim light of injustice and bad breaks. However, there is way around this.

Video games have drawn adults back into the world of make-believe, with role-playing games that take us to faraway lands, sometimes in the body of a different being altogether. In daily life, we use the imagination regularly to empathize with someone else's circumstances and feelings. Only a human being can detach from his or her own situation and perceive, albeit in a limited way, what it is like to walk in someone else's shoes. This ability is what we will use now in the following exercise that is sure to tap into the true goodness of your life.

For those days when you can't feel any good in your life or when some problem is looming, obscuring your view, the following tool can be invaluable to break through and see your life and world through the eyes of another person. But who should that imaginary person be? Well, believe it or not, it should be you! I will show you how to go back in time to when you were just a kid and then allow the present version of yourself to come and show you all the amazing things you will have in your life. Things you take for granted, such as your home, loved ones, past achievements, and the way others perceive you. But now you will be able to see everything in your life with fresh eyes. When you stand as that younger version of yourself listening to all of the wonderful things you will have in your future, it will be easy to see how far you have come in your life and in your development.

This exercise is particularly helpful if you are struggling with a lot of anxiety because this mental separation disengages all of the judgment filters that you normally force all information through. Until these filters are dissolved, it can be difficult some days to see your life in a positive light. It is as though you are standing in a courtroom trying to convince a jury that your life has some great things in it when the prosecutor suddenly jumps up and yells, "Objection, Your Honor; this is hearsay and can't be proven!" Yeah, we all have that guy in our head from time to time.

This practice will allow you to be as receptive as a wide-eyed child. Your brain underestimates your past accomplishments and achievements just as it does with many of your present ones. But this method of having someone else tell you about your achievements will allow you to revisit these facts and feel how monumental they really are. Make sure that you hear and see this imaginary version of you; make it as real as you can, and take your time.

Back in Time Exercise:

Click here for a link to an audible version of the following visualization.

Close your eyes and take four long breaths. See yourself at a younger age somewhere between nine and thirteen years old. Then feel yourself as that young person and see yourself comfortably sitting somewhere, curiously wondering what your future holds. Let that time come back to you as strongly as possible. Allow yourself to travel back there, hearing all the sounds and feeling all the feelings you felt back then. Then this person, (an older version of yourself) walks up to you, smiles, and sits down next to you. They look familiar, and as you try to understand what is happening. They look at you and say, I'm here to give you a little peek into your future, would you like that? You nod as they seem very familiar to you. They begin telling you about all the things you will have in the future at your current age. They tell you about every good thing you have (house, car, family, friends, mate, job, etc.). You stand up together, and they begin taking you around your home showing you the things you own, the car you drive, the clothes you wear, your pets, and your best friends. Listen carefully, hearing this as a child would be for the first time. What it is like to use a phone with no wires, to read the news off a screen that is not a TV and to type on a keyboard with no paper instead your words appear on that same screen. They try to describe what the Internet is and a tablet. You hear about how big TV's are and what a home theater is. You are in awe as you listen to how you will be able connect to your childhood friends through something called Facebook and send letters to friends thousands of miles away in only seconds. You are spellbound as you listen to this older version of you describe how you have overcome different trials and are stronger for it. You are amazed at how many people count on you for help and even their survival. You can do this out loud, in a whisper, or in your head. A whisper can to be very helpful as long as you do it in second person. Feel the amazement that comes over you. You know it's working when a smile comes across your face. Many people can't believe how well this technique works. It's because doing this in the second person removes the subjective, critical judge. This allows you to really accept all the good things happening in your life without judging yourself or feeling guilty about them. When done answer the following questions.

On a scale of one to ten, how powerful was this for you? _____

_____

Of the things you normally take for granted, what touched you the most?

_____

What part of your life made you feel the best?

_____

_____

Did anything come to mind that surprised you?

_____

_____

Did you remember anything about your current life as you did this exercise that you forgot made an impact on who you have become?

_____

_____

What amazing things came to mind that you have overcome?

_____

_____

Did you feel more gratitude towards your family and friends than you are normally aware of?

_____

_____

Can you see how even current technology is something to feel very grateful for?

_____

_____

Note if you felt safer, more hopeful, or inspired. Describe.

_____

_____

_____

_____

_____

13

USING GOOD MEMORIES TO ERASE PAST PAIN

AS I HAVE BEEN SAYING YOUR MEMORY PLAYS AN INTEGRAL ROLE IN BRINGING BACK BOTH GOOD AND BAD EVENTS FOR YOU TO RELIVE. These memories don't even have to be factual because your brain is not concerned with how memories are formed—whether you were awake, just dreaming, or mistakenly distorted a childhood event. If it happened in your mind, it happened. Even a forgotten or buried memory can still wield great influence over your actions. For instance, you can glance across a crowded room and immediately dislike someone because your brain determines he looks or sounds like someone else you didn't like. From that point forward, that individual will have a snowball's chance in hell of hitting it off with you.

Overriding Painful Memories with Positive Ones

You have spent your whole life building strong memories of times when you were hurt, allowing them to evolve into perceptions about people, places or things. We do this to protect ourselves from similar future situations. Now your brain will be doing the same thing with your new positive experiences, even retracing old positive events in your mind and making them easy to recall as well, like you have been practicing in the previous exercises.

Another very powerful way to use these memories is to attach them to old negative ones, to fears, and even to some phobias. Again, we are just using the power of your imagination.

Let me illustrate this. I had a client, a very attractive young girl in her twenties. She was confident, outgoing, and intelligent, but she had a recurring issue of becoming very nervous and self-conscious anytime she had to walk into a building by herself. There seemed to be no event in her past to trigger this kind of fear. One of the places the fear seemed to affect her was yoga class. She loved attending yoga, but she often struggled at the thought of walking in alone and would wait for other people to walk in first. Sitting in her car trying to analyze it while trying to get up the courage to walk in by herself was becoming daunting and frustrating. So we utilized this technique to overwrite her fear using something she enjoyed doing.

Because my client loved yoga, we started by having her visualize herself enjoying a yoga class. It took only a moment of visualizing the class with its smells and sounds for her to feel it deeply. Then I coached her to slowly allow the memory and thought of walking into the yoga school by herself to come up. When she felt the nervousness come in, she immediately went back to the thought of being in the yoga class enjoying herself. She did this back and forth between visualizations for about five minutes. During the week, she applied this same technique while in the yoga class. When she felt peaceful and contented, she would picture herself walking into the school; when she felt the nervousness, she would bring herself back to the present moment in the class. What was magically happening was that she was allowing her brain to wire these two events together. Walking into yoga class by herself was now attached to the wonderful feelings she experienced in the yoga class. Within a week, she was walking into the school by herself. She allowed her enjoyment of doing yoga to erase the nervousness and awkwardness; her brain now associated the walking into the building only with her pure enjoyment of yoga. She also applied this to other destinations where she had to walk in by herself, connecting them to the same memory of doing yoga and feeling wonderful, and it worked for those as well. Remember, **what fires together wires together**.

Once I had a client who had a fear of public speaking, which was a real problem because she wanted to do this regularly. She taught people how to train their dogs, and over the years she had received a mountain of thank-you cards from very grateful clients. In one of our visualizations, I had her imagine being onstage feeling the nervousness and then imagine having all of those people there standing up to read their thank-you note to her. She would allow herself to feel the nervousness but only in the background while also feeling elated at all the gratitude being shown to her. She practiced this several times over two days, associating her first nervous moments onstage with grateful clients in front of her giving her all kinds of accolades. Her first minute onstage was the hardest, so this proved to get her over the initial hump.

In utilizing good memories or positive current experiences to help you override something negative, you need to look for positive issues that are specific to the same family of negative material, using the categories you learned earlier. For example, an experience of a friend who hurt you would be countered with memories of the good solid friends you also have in your life. Just recalling these emotions is all you need because your brain has no idea whether it is happening now or just in your imagination.

First let's fill your toolbox with some great memories that you can pull up fast and easy. I want you to try to recall some past great experiences to feel their good all over again just as you did with your vacation memory. Take your time, at least ten seconds, for each one.

Use Memories and Imagination to Feel Good Right Now

- The memory of a child giving you a hug or a kiss.
- The memory of a puppy licking your face.
- The memory of eating the most delicious desert.
- The memory of sitting with the sun warming your body on a beautiful but chilly summer day.
- The memory of a really funny story.
- The feeling of unwrapping a Christmas or birthday present.
- The memory of purchasing a big luxury item, such as a house, car, or home theater.
- A memory of your young child wrapping their arms around your neck and saying, "I love you".
- The memory of you making others laugh.
- The memory of someone saying "You helped me so much"

List Ten Wonderful Memories of Your Own:

1 _____

2 _____

3 _____

4 _____

5 _____

6 _____

7 _____

8 _____

9 _____

10 _____

Now we are going to use these memories to effectively override the pain associated with some old negative memories. For the best and fastest results, be sure the good memories closely relate to the discomfort you are feeling.

To do this, you will identify the root emotion you want to override so you can counter it effectively. At first it will take some practice to discern what triggers your emotions; you may well believe it is one thing but discover it was something else. So if you have memories of being unappreciated and taken for granted but assume it's just a feeling of loneliness, then thinking of times when you were around friends having fun and laughter will not be that helpful. You would instead need to remember times of being appreciated, valued, and recognized. The key is to be clear on what your **beliefs** are about these memories.

Write down a painful emotion then under that the antidote (happy memory)

1 _____

_____

2 _____

_____

3 _____

_____

4 _____

_____

Rewiring the Anxiety Circuit

Several summers ago, I had been experiencing some chronic anxiety that seemed to persist under most of my daily activities. Even though I was not depressed, no matter what thought came to mind, it triggered a sense of anxiety and dread. I went on vacation to the Jersey Shore and had been doing some journaling at the beach when I had an epiphany. For those of you who don't know, I make various kinds of art. Suddenly, I realized my best piece of art work is still ahead of me. This ignited me. I had no idea that I had been doubting my skills and my ability to come up with another really outstanding painting. Subconsciously, for whatever reason, I was under the impression that my best artwork was behind me after applying myself for only about eight years! Why? Did I think that was the lifetime of an artist? Of course not; the fact was, I was only getting started, and I knew that was a truth I could trust.

The following day when I felt the anxiety, I immediately repeated out loud, "My best artwork is ahead of me." I waited and made sure I felt the same elation I had felt the day before. The anxiety dissipated! I froze right where I stood. Was it a fluke or coincidence? Moments later, I tried it again and felt happy with no anxiety. Throughout the day, I then continued to bring this truth back to mind with all of its feeling each time I felt the slightest wave of anxiety, which at that point was happening several times an hour. I would simply say out loud, "My best artwork is ahead of me," and the anxiety would vanish!

What happened next though really surprised me. In only two days, when something occurred that would normally trigger an anxious feeling, my brain automatically triggered the great feelings I'd had about making my best piece of artwork! Not the thought, just the wonderful emotions were on the heels of every anxious thought I had! This blew me away. My brain somehow had associated my negative thoughts with positive emotions! The brain is very efficient; once it recognized that I brought up my art at the onset of any anxiety, it simply began to release the good, happy feelings before I even had a chance to recite the thought to trigger them. I didn't need to recall the thought about making art anymore!

I couldn't help but be amazed; as any concern that crossed my mind immediately brought this wave of happiness. Much later, I bought Rick Hansen's book "Hardwiring Happiness" and read his detailed description of this process. It confirmed this wasn't some kind of fluke but rather was a real, repeatable skill. I then realized that I could duplicate this same experience with a host of past emotions as well, not just present ones.

Many years ago before that experience, I was working at a client's office 8 hours every Friday. It was unrelated to my normal field of expertise. I disliked the work and this client. After 3 months on a Thursday I found myself really dreading the next day. So that Friday after she handed me my usual pay. I spent time looking at it, thinking of what I would buy, how nice it was to be flush with money. I felt it, smelled it and waited until I could feel the pleasure down to my toes. From that moment forward every time I thought about spending Friday there, I immediately thought about the feeling of getting the money and what it would be like. I was always dreading this place, so I was doing this practice several times a day but in only a couple of days I had permanently linked the good feelings about the money with the thought of going. I stopped hating Fridays! I had no idea about this rewiring my brain or that I could repeat this practice back then and it still worked wonderfully. Since then I have done this countless times with any experience I am dreading from a dentist visit, to preparing myself to sit in traffic.

Using this technique to over ride bad memories is the next

step you will practice. I can't overstate the power and usefulness of this as it has changed the lives of countless clients. You will be amazed by how different bad memories will feel as their sting dissipates.

Doing the steps below several times a day will allow your brain to automatically tie positive emotions to negative memories. This is the beauty of neuroplasticity!

The Technique

You override one feeling with another by holding two thoughts in your mind the way my clients did in the previous stories. Make sure the positive thought or fact relates to the category of the negative memory. Holding two thoughts at the same time is like raising the volume on the TV (the positive memories) to drown out the loud voices in the background (the negative memories). You hear both, but you focus only on the TV.

Let's begin by relieving negative emotions you may experience when you have to do annoying tasks. Pick a particular task that bugs you. Nothing major for now, just something that bugs you at between a three and five on a scale of one to ten. Could be folding clothes, taking out the garbage, or doing something at work. Try to identify why it bugs you: it is boring, it lacks importance, or you feel under-valued when doing it. Then come up with a great memory that makes you feel the opposite.

Now to counteract a feeling of being lonely or rejected, thinking of your vacation spot would not be appropriate. You need to think of a correlating positive memory. Take the good memory and let it resonate within you. Let it be vivid and bright, until you feel it sinking into every cell and then gradually allow the annoying task to come to mind. When you feel frustrated, let it slip back into the background while you feel the good memory, Do this several times. The exact result can be different for each person, but most can rewire themselves to feel good about whatever annoyed them in one day. After a full day of this, you will notice that your brain will begin to go right to the good memory before you can even feel annoyed. Your brain has tied the two experiences together.

As an example, two men drive a bus for a living. When you ask Driver 1 how he likes it, he says, "I hate it. Driving in NYC traffic all day is hell, the people are rude, and it is stressful." When Driver 2 is asked the same question, he says, "What I like about it is what it provides for me. It gives me a way to have a steady income for my family. Every time I am stuck in traffic, I think of how I am being paid just to sit there, and I plan what that money will buy for my kids. I also think about how all these people are counting on me to do my job right so they can do theirs." He used these truths to radiate positive feelings whenever he encountered things he didn't like, thereby teaching his brain to trigger feel-good chemicals when these things took place. This has much to do with perspective, but what is fascinating is that the brain can quickly initiate the good feelings once it sees the pattern you are generating, causing it to become a natural state. This is the training; this is the rewiring.

Attaching a Past Memory to the Present Annoyance of a Child

Here is something to do if you are a parent with a child who does something that bugs you (nothing really serious but rather a pet peeve). On the next page, write the memory of when the child was born and how it felt to hold him or her in your arms for the first time. Write out each detail. Try to recall every thought that went through your mind about this child and his or her future. You want to recapture all of the emotion of that moment. Stay with it until it is very strong with great detail.

Now, while that memory is really vivid in your mind with all the emotion, allow the thought of what the child does to be in the background. When you feel a small amount of frustration rising, bring back the memory of when he or she was born. Do this repeatedly until you feel only the emotion of the birth when you think of his or her annoying habit.

You can do this with your spouse as well, using the memory of your wedding day or the day you got engaged or recounting how you met.

_____

_____

_____

_____

Attaching a Future Memory to a Present Annoyance of Child

There is a second way for you parents to ease your frustration when you have a child who is lacking in some kind of maturity. Here we will use your imagination of the future to your advantage. Imagine your child on his or her wedding day. Envision it with all the details you can. Bring in every emotion of happiness, pride, and hope that you will have that day, and write it below. Do this two or three times to solidify it.

Once the visualization is very strong, write it out and then sit with it. Very gradually allow the memory of the child's present behavior to creep in. When you feel angry or frustrated, bring the wedding scene to the forefront. Do this until you feel your brain releasing the good feelings at the thought of the annoying behavior.

_____

_____

_____

_____

_____

_____

_____

_____

_____

Recalling Specific Types of Memories

First come up with your three happiest memories that made you feel loved, adored, special, appreciated, and included. Write down as many details as you can.

Write out the following answers by recalling each one with great detail. Once you have done that sit with each one and recall every emotional detail you can. (Do not attempt these if you are in PMS or are particularly stressed out)

1) Think of three past situations with a loved one that made you feel special, unique, and valued.

_____

_____

_____

_____

_____

_____

_____

_____

_____

_____

_____

_____

_____

_____

_____

2) Think back to when you were in school when a teacher or other authority made you feel smart, gifted, or special in any way.

_____

_____

_____

_____

_____

_____

3) Think of a time when a boss or superior complimented your efforts on a task or overall performance.

_____

_____

_____

_____

4) Describe the most beautiful thing you ever saw or experienced.

_____

_____

_____

_____

_____

Now name a painful memory at least five years old of when you felt ignored, left out, or unappreciated. No need for details here. Just name it.

Now for the next thirty seconds, all I want you to do is feel one of the best memories you wrote. Make sure it is a powerful memory of love and appreciation. Wait until you can feel yourself smiling, soaking in the actual emotion of that moment. If you aren't smiling, it may not be strong or vivid enough. Now very gently allow the negative memory to be in the background, just like loud voices you are drowning out with a TV. Be aware of both. When you can feel the sting of the negative one, go right back to the happy one. Continue to bounce between them for two minutes. Then open your eyes.

Doing this practice for two to three minutes about five to seven times a day will create an association so that your brain will automatically release your feel-good neurotransmitters every time the negative memory resurfaces! Most people get results after one day.

An even more powerful way to do this is to wait until you are having a tremendously warm, wonderful experience, maybe with a niece, nephew, grandchild, or new puppy. It should be something special, loving, and lighthearted. Once you are fully present to all the warmth and love of that moment, begin to allow an old painful memory to surface, but only in the background, When you feel its sting, come back to the present moment, feeling all of the love and warmth of being with the kids or a pet. Do this several times until all you feel are great emotions even when the old memory is present. You have replaced the old negative emotion with the new positive one. You just rewired your mind!

I will mention here that these are not a replacement for working directly with a therapist with whom you discuss painful childhood memories. By bringing these painful memories to light in the safety of the office with a caring therapist, your mind will begin a new kind of emotional association with the memory, using the same principle of connecting positive with negative.

Erase the negative emotions with the new positive feelings.

List five past events that trigger pain that you would like to erase.

No need for details just list them.

1 _____

2 _____

3 _____

4 _____

5 _____

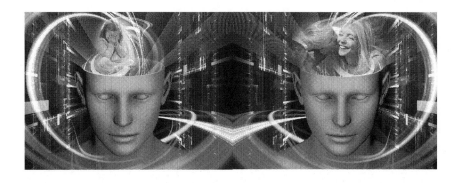

USE THE COLUMNS BELOW TO LIST THE
NEGATIVE MEMORIES WITH THE POSITIVE ONES

Painful Memories	Happy Memories

14

LAST THOUGHTS

WE NEED TO BE AWARE THAT IF WE ARE GOING WITHOUT SLEEP OR EATING SUGARY, HIGH-CARBOHYDRATE MEALS, WE ARE CHEMICALLY SETTING OURSELVES UP FOR MOOD SWINGS.

If you eat a sugary lunch or don't lunch at all, by three o'clock you will not be on your toes, aware, and alert. You will fall asleep at the wheel, and the old program will take over. Your expectations will be there, disappointment will occur, and you will personalize everything that goes wrong simply because your mind is too dull to catch these mental shifts before they happen. Make no mistake about it—we are still not much different from overtired toddlers; we just have more self-discipline. (OK, a little more.)

When I first began to apply these techniques and new way of thinking, I would become complacent at times. Things would be running so smoothly that I would forget to pause every couple of hours to feel the good around me, or I would allow my mind to wander down the road a bit to the next thing I wanted to accomplish. Then suddenly something would go wrong, and I would be caught off guard. I would find myself getting angry all because I forgot to pay attention to what was happening in the moment and had not soaked my brain in the happy juices of DOS. Happily, I can report that due to neuroplasticity, my brain is now doing many of these techniques automatically without my conscious brain having to remind me. I just naturally find myself constantly taking in good things, and if I find I am thinking about the past or future, my mind automatically pulls me back to the present. Your brain, too, will begin to rewire permanently. It just takes some consistent awareness. The best practice is always to start your day with the mindfulness meditation and at the end of your day write in your journal what you are grateful for. During the day keep a mental check list of what expectations you might be setting yourself up for. Remember whatever happens—it isn't personal!

Handling High Anxiety

When that really crummy day happens and you find you let yourself become anxious, the neurochemicals that work best to calm it down are endorphins and oxytocin. Anxiety makes it really hard to experience serotonin and dopamine. Studies have shown that oxytocin and endorphins are best for triggering relaxation and calm. Is it any wonder we are wired to get the fastest dose of oxytocin from our partner? I guess evolution understood marriage could be tough at times.

To get a big dose of endorphins or oxytocin, have a great night of sex, cuddle with someone you love, sit with an infant, or spend time nurturing your children. Even being with your pet or volunteering at an animal shelter can do wonders. The most consistent way is get to the gym for some aerobic exercise (at least thirty minutes, if you are healthy enough); I don't mean to be repetitive but it is safer and works more efficiently than any drug we have on the market. Do an intense or endurance sport such as skiing, jet skiing, running, snowboarding, or biking. Research has even found that sunbathing can release endorphins; that is why a day at the beach can rejuvenate almost anyone and why tanning can be addicting. The majority of the people I meet at my gym who are over forty claim that the main reason they exercise is for the emotional benefits—even more than for physical conditioning. **Exercise done right can get you out of a state of anxiety and keep you out for forty-eight to seventy-two hours. Guaranteed. No drug can promise that.**

Whom can you nurture?

_____

With whom can you cuddle?

_____

Who makes you feel really safe and cared for?

_____

Who gives the best hugs?

_____

What sport or exercise could you take up?

_____

Your Progression

After about three weeks of recalling good memories and seeing and feeling all the good around you regularly, you will find that your tolerance for problems, disappointments, and setbacks has increased. When a bill arrives or your boss has an attitude, your brain will naturally recall these things of comfort before you go into fight-and-protect mode, and you will immediately feel a sense of relief and safety. When you notice that you are reacting to a situation out of habit, you will be able to feel that the emotion is not nearly as strong as it used to be. Your reaction will now be calmer because of the extra supply of DOS you now carry.

After I was 5 weeks into a regular practice of this training I remember seeing a parking space and as I approached, out of nowhere a car pulled into it right in front of me. I had my blinker on, so I believed it was deliberate. I instantly let out some choice words, but then I stopped and had to chuckle. I wasn't feeling the anger that normally would have accompanied such language. I was reacting out of pure habit, and truthfully, I really didn't feel anything about it. I wondered, "Hold on; is this real?" I was amazed. I had been making an effort to feel appreciative all day, so this little blip didn't even register on my radar. Yes, I had to battle my old thought patterns—that out of pure principle, I should say something—but now that was a choice, and I chose to just keep feeling happy.

When your amygdala goes off unexpectedly and determines that a situation warrants anxiety or fear, it will be a challenge to start trying to allow the good around you to soak in. At times you may notice your brain going into crisis mode while your mind tries like hell to think its way out of it and find good things around you. However, trying to feel them after you are in crisis mode will be hard. The cortisol and adrenaline are overriding everything at that point. **When it comes to these hormones, it's first come, first served.**

Keep your brain swimming in good feelings; then, when a situation does arise, the DOS chemicals will win out. Remember the analogy of keeping logs wet so that the panic fires can't start. Keeping your brain soaked in dopamine, oxytocin, and serotonin will keep the other neurochemicals, cortisol and adrenaline, from being able to wreak havoc. This is your goal!

After reading this book and faithfully practicing your exercises, you will notice changes in the first week. Annoyances from another driver, a derogatory comment, or a family member requiring more than you have to give will sting much less. You will notice how you start reminding yourself of everything that you have learned. After one or two days, this constant choice to remember that you now *have a choice* is the first step, and although you may not experience happiness or bliss in the first two or three days, you will begin feeling a sense of relief that you are not forced to react. **The rewiring has already started.**

By the fourth day, of consistently taking in the good around you, you will begin to feel some relief, a sense of hope around this new pattern of thinking developing.

In days 5-7, you will be maintaining a calmer demeanor. You will be less afraid of uncomfortable situations. You will begin to notice that problems are working out without you getting worked up.

In week 2, you will be able to bring up good feelings over past or present facts and events more quickly. You will smile more, and although no specific event is occurring, you will have a stronger sense of well-being. You should feel more approachable.

By week 3 frustrating situations should bring only the memories of the old reactions. You may find yourself uttering the same verbal retort or sarcasm, just as I did when I lost my parking space, but you will notice that the old negative emotions are not there nearly as strong as they were before.

After 60 days, most report that they are happier, more easygoing, and more hopeful about their future than ever before. No longer living in fear of the next crisis, they have a sense of strength confidence and stability

You will take great pleasure in affecting your environment; people will begin to relate differently to you because you will be operating out of this base of security, confidence, and safety, and they will notice the change. You just need to commit for one month. Just one month for about thirty minutes a day, including meditation time, and your mind will rewire itself! I know you are busy, but most of that busyness is rooted in trying to find the sweet spot of peace. If you are reading this, I know that much of your time is consumed with being stressed and unhappy. You have to decide once and for all—do you want more than anything to wake up with a sense of peace and well-being? Or would you rather continue commiserating with everyone around you ruminating about future events that haven't even occurred yet? Don't you want to recapture and maintain the feeling you have while on vacation? Isn't it worthwhile to sit quietly when everyone starts ranting about our government leaders, knowing you can wake up with a smile? How desperate are you?

I was desperate. I finally decided I no longer wanted to live opening my eyes each morning and not being sure what mood I would be in and then have it affect me all day. Even waking up in a good mood for no reason was frustrating because I didn't know what to do to harness it. Nothing had changed in my life—not a darn thing—but there it was, calm peace of mind! I knew there had to be a way to harness that magic. Well it's here. The hardest part will be your commitment; the process is very straightforward. It's up to you. Finding happiness is the motive behind every action, behavior, thought, and idea we concoct. So just do it already!

Sign up in our Facebook Group for the readers of this book (Get Off Your Worry-Go-Round)and say, "I'm in; I want to feel happy." Talk with others and enjoy the inspiration and encouragement from those who want to make the most of their lives. And remember, none of us lives in a vacuum; everything we do affects those around us. Whom will you help?

From now on, your job is to spread the word that we really do have a choice about how to feel. We can choose to feel good now and stay present or chase some elusive promise that we will feel good later, when all our problems are handled—which never happens!

Remember These Rules:

1) Your brain, has a broken outdated warning system.

2) Stop taking life personally and waiting for the lottery.

3) Find good things around you every hour and feel them for 10 sec. Remember **FEEL** them, not just notice them!

4) Keep your brain soaked in DOS to ward off the effects of your overreactive amygdala.

5) Never leave your mind unattended on autopilot; if you do, it will rush into the future or back into the past. Only you can take it to those places safely.

On the following pages, I list actions and their correlating neurotransmitter release. These can vary, depending on your prior experiences. Also, your propensity toward a particular chemical is due to thousands of experiences you have had over the course of your life. Some experiences may have been on purpose and others accidental, but either way, they molded you to seek out certain experiences that you feel are good for you.

All of the neurochemicals I discuss in this book are complex in terms of how they do what they do; they are all tied to various other chemicals in the mind and body. In no way am I trying to oversimplify their functions. Even science is only beginning to understand them. I wrote this book only to give you a basic comprehension to the degree that it can help you live a happier and more fulfilled life. I did not intend for this book to be a scientific reference, however, I wrote it using only verified scientific studies and documentation from the most qualified scientific journals. I purposely chose not overwhelm readers with these references as this book was written for the lay person who just wants to FEEL BETTER. I will at some point however be including these on my website.

Please continue to learn about your brain; the story is only just beginning to unfold, thanks to technology.

Soon it will be a thing of the past for doctors to try to guess what their patients need for depression, ADHD, or bipolar disorder. In the next five years, you will see an explosion of information coming out about that three-pound mass above your shoulders. Researchers will know the root causes of mental disorders and will be able to alter them with a more direct approach. If you suffer from a serious mental illness, please hang in there; help is coming. In no way are the ideas in this book meant to minimize the suffering associated with serious mental illness or to take the place of professional medical help. There are chemical alterations in the brain that only medical intervention can address. I know all too well there is no illness on earth as painful as mental illness. My hope is that eventually self-help groups will become mainstream for those suffering so that at least the isolation can be minimized. I am living proof that spontaneous alterations in the brain can happen; as it happened to me in 1996. PLEASE DO NOT GIVE UP. We are finally getting close to some real answers.

DOPAMINE

BEHAVIORS LINKED TO OUR SURVIVAL INSTINCTS

We argue our point.	We compete.
We attend sporting events.	We pursue sexual partners.
We play video games.	We enjoy concerts.
We fight.	We challenge authority
We fall in love.	We go out dancing.
We go out to dinner.	We play competitive sports.
We strive for promotions	We push our kids to excel.
We participate in illegal activity.	We gamble.
We challenge the opinions of others.	We play the stock market.
We surf, ski, or skateboard.	We like action movies.
We remodel our home.	We enjoy fast vehicles.
We rant about injustice.	We like scavenger hunts.
We love traveling to new places.	We plan vacations.
We pledge to college Frat or Sorority.	We argue our point.
We sing along with a song.	We ride roller coasters.
We complain.	We explode.
We do speed drugs and diet pills.	We cheer for our teams.
We overindulge in caffeine.	We ride motorcycles.

More Details on Dopamine

Many people like to describe an elevation in dopamine as "motivation" or "pleasure." But that's too simple. Actually, dopamine signals feedback for anticipated rewards. However dopamine doesn't only predict rewards; It actually tells the brain to pay attention and focus on something, and when you obey your brain, it begins to reward you.

SEROTONIN

BEHAVIORS LINKED TO OUR SURVIVAL INSTINCTS

We seek for status at work.	We give blood.
We buy second homes in beautiful places.	We seek and hope for mates who are better than we are.
We wear our team's logo.	We help others.
We safeguard our home.	We challenge others.
We fall in love with those we perceive as better than ourselves.	We gush with pride about our children.
We brag.	We want the spot light.
We strive for better bodies.	We go on vacation.
We photograph things of beauty.	We associate with celebrities.
We make friends with others who have high social status or are rich.	We post our good times on Facebook.
We throw parties.	We try to be funny.
We learn a new language.	We protect our beliefs.
We go out to fancy restaurants	We volunteer.
We buy expensive clothing.	We monopolize conversations
We learn to play an instrument.	We are better at talking than listening

Oxytocin

Behaviors Linked to Our Survival Instincts

We hold hands.	We laugh together.
We hug.	We play with our pets.
We play with children.	We provide for our children
We caress.	We get massages.
We compliment each other.	We rescue animals.
We have sex.	We kiss.
We join gangs.	We cook for those we love.
We join groups.	We include others.
We mentor a young person.	We let others win.
We choose to be around those with similar problems, likes or beliefs like drinking or drugs, disabilities, illness, race.	We try to make each other laugh.

ALL 3 DOS EVENTS

THESE COULD TARGET ALL 3 NEUROCHEMICALS
(PLUS SOME ENDORPHINS),
MAKING PEOPLE VERY PASSIONATE ABOUT THEM.

Going to church.

Joining a political party.

Running a successful fund drive.

Being at the stadium as your team wins a championship.

Speaking or performing well on stage.

Hosting an event.

Having a baby.

Saving a life.

Hitting a home run or scoring a goal.

Having sex when you are madly in love.

Getting married.

Being proposed to.

On the following pages are some detailed disappointments that can sometimes trigger a decrease in a specific neurochemical. It helps to know this when you want to relieve that feeling. However, again each person is different and various experiences may mean very different things to different readers. So this is just a guide to help you figure out yourself.

EXPERIENCES THAT
CAN CAUSE A DIP IN YOUR DOPAMINE

- Going to your favorite restaurant only to find it closed.

- Going into the freezer to dig out some ice cream to find it gone.

- Going to a store for a sale to find that the sale is over or there is nothing left.

- Trying to make the light only to have it turn red before you get there.

- Going to the movies and finding yours is sold out.

- Losing in any competition,from board games, to street racing.

- Seeing a potential lover across the room only to see that he or she is with someone.

- Losing at the craps table, slots or lottery.

- Being picked for the losing team.

- Having your political candidate lose.

- Realizing you can't afford something.

- Finding a long line in any restaurant or coffee shop.

- Regretting having bought an expensive item.

- Encountering delay in any kind of gratification.

The old cliché "The thrill of the chase is better than the catch" was a profound observation considering they had no idea dopamine even existed and why women were admonished to "play hard to get" with possible suitors.

Experiences That Can Cause a
Dip In Your Oxytocin

- Being ill and not having human comfort.

- Being deprived of contact with your lover.

- Not being hugged, touched or kissed.

- Not having sex.

- Being cooped up in your house due to weather (having no social contact)

- Having a week in which everything seems to go wrong.

- Reaching out to friends via phone or Internet and not getting a response.

- Having your child refuse to connect with you.

- Having your spouse or lover reject your advances.

- Being told you can't join a group or organization.

Experiences That Can Cause a Dip In Your Serotonin

- Being around people who like to show everyone how much money they have or vacations they go on or the home improvements they have made.

- Your superior telling you that you need to improve.

- Another co-worker getting accolades or a raise. (This makes things so uncomfortable as we really want to feel "happy" for them but we can't but help but feel crummy inside due to the serotonin drop.)

- Saying something dumb in public.(The fear of public speaking is ranked as the #1 fear, because to publically fail or be humiliated would mean a gross depletion of serotonin and although it poses no physical harm your amygdala screams "don't do it.!"

- Being around happy couples if you are single.

- In America you can feel your serotonin drop just from watching TV because marketers have mastered the art of making you feel "less than". "Unless you have-- (insert product) you will not be be safe, secure and superior to others". Although they don't use those words, I just wish once a comercial aired with the real meaning running under it in subtitles, "You suck unless you drive this!" "Your friends will laugh at your yellow teeth!"

- Experiencing anything that threatens your safety: car breaking down, feeling sick, thinking others are talking about you.

- Not having the money to buy something in the moment.

- People interrupting or talking over you in a conversation.

- Experiencing a threat to your financial security.

- A bill, higher interest rates, things breaking down from your car to appliances, losing your wallet, kids needing this or that. All of this can swing your mood very fast. It will feel like death to your brain but it isn't, so don't agree with the feeling.

- Although we know we are not perfect, when others confront us about our mistakes or character flaws, we often argue or redirect attention because the dip in our serotonin levels feels so horrible. But being able to admit to faults or failures breeds trust. In the long run, our serotonin will soar when we sense the respect that we receive for doing so.

ABOUT THE AUTHOR

PUBLIC SPEAKER, EDUCATOR. COUNSELOR, TRAINER, AUTHOR AND ARTIST, Sharie is a philosopher, a visionary, a riot, a role model and a beacon of light for those in the throws of mental darkness.

Sharie has an unquenchable thirst not only to learn about neuropsychology (how the brain makes us tick) but also to teach it to others and has been doing so since 1985. In the '80s, she was a highly sought motivational speaker who taught at high schools and colleges. Both the kids and psychology professors gained new insight about themselves using science, wisdom, and experience.

In 1986, she co-produced the David Toma show on WOR for a year, working closely with David to reach teens on an international level. She then spearheaded and became the director of the David Toma Center in Tecate, Mexico, a rehabilitation center for those caught up in drugs and alcohol.

Sharie was at the top of her field as an educator, therapist and motivational spokesperson when her world suddenly fell apart. After she was diagnosed with rapid cycling bipolar depression in 1990, her life came to a crashing halt. For the next six years, Sharie's journey in and out of hospitals left her hopeless, tired, and ready to quit. Despite her unending research of this disorder, the twenty-one doctors she saw were unable to prescribe anything that would give her stability for longer than a few weeks.

Between March 31 and April 3, 1996, just before she gave up, a miracle transpired, and Sharie was radically healed of any and all mood swings after having an 86 year old women name Fuchsia Pickett pray for her over the course of 4 nights. When she reported to her doctor, he told her that what had happened was impossible. She left his office smiling from ear to ear; his disbelief made what happened to her even more profound. This propelled Sharie to discover how the miracle happened and whether a scientific explanation existed as well as God's divine intervention. It was in 1996 that neuroplasticity was confirmed, proving that the human brain can change and heal itself.

Sharie has a deep passion to reach into the human soul and grab hold of what matters to people. She is not afraid to use her incredible past to inspire others. Sharie has a gift for explaining technical, scientific details, using humor, metaphors, and pure wisdom. Through techniques based on neuroscience and using ten seconds at a time, she can help you rewire your brain for happiness and learn about you.

Sharie is available for workshops, readings, one-on-one sessions, and speaking engagements.

Contact Info
www.shariespironhi.com

Social Media Connections

www.facebook.com 10secondstohappy

https://itunes.apple.com/us/podcast/
10-seconds-to-happys-podcast

http://TenSecondsToHappy.podbean.com

http://twitter.com/SharieSpironhi

Help make this book even better.
If you have any ideas or suggestions please email them for review. I will add any helpful ideas to the next edition. As well as put them on the my website.

ADDITIONAL RESOURCES

Below are some excellent books that paved the way for this book to be written. Also the following websites will give you clear understandings about mindfulness and mediation and expedite your learning.

http://www.meditationsecretsrevealed.com
http://www.mindful.org/mindfulness-practice

Stress-Proof Your Brain: Meditations to Rewire Neural Pathways for Stress Relief and Unconditional Happiness 2010, by Ph. D Rick Hanson
Hardwiring Happiness: The New Brain Science of Contentment Calm, and Confidence 2013 by Rick Hanson

The Scientific American Book of Love, Sex and the Brain:
The Neuroscience of How, When, Why and Who We Love
2011 by Judith Horstman

The Female Brain: 2007, by Louann Brizendine
The Male Brain: 2011, by Louann Brizendine

The Power of Now : A Guide to Spiritual Enlightenment
A New Heaven and a New Earth: Awakening to Your Life's Purpose
by Eckart Tolle

Finding Flow: The Psychology of Engagement with Everyday Life
1997, by Mihaly Csikszentmihalyi

The Brain that Changes Itself. 2007, by Norman Doidge, MD

The Message of You Book & The Message of You Journal:
Finding Extraordinary Stories in an Ordinary Day 2015, by Judy Carter

The Power of Intention. 2005, by Wayne Dyer

ACKNOWLEDGMENTS

This section could be a book in itself if I were to name every person who has helped me along my journey. Books such as this one are not written overnight but rather evolve over years within the soul of the writer. This accumulation of understanding, wisdom, and guidance was birthed only this past year but was conceived many years ago.

There is often that pivotal moment, a divine appointment, when your path crosses with that of another, setting the stage for a course correction. I have had many of those, but one of the most recent individuals who helped to launch this phase of my life was Judy Carter, who confirmed that I had a message people would want to hear on many levels and showed me how to begin digging to find it. Thank you for lighting the fuse! The other person was Cynthia Malaran, who got me talking about all of this so it began to take shape. Your enthusiasm and confidence got my pen moving.

Thanks to Sarah Douma Schweighardt, who didn't hesitate to lend her brilliance, time and energy for the first draft reads. Your support for this book's potential kept me going. Now please finish yours!

For Carole DeLaOsa and Dr. Margret Karsky-Zaffarese, who jumped in with wide eyed enthusiasm. Your ideas, suggestions, and encouragement were invaluable.

To all the people who gave me feedback on the endless cover renditions. Your insight and ideas helped me define what I wanted to say.

To the first group of people who sat through my workshop Duane, Esther, Yvonne, Mary, Debbie. Your excitement and interest quickly helped me realize that I had to write this book.

My life proved to be the classroom that would teach me everything I needed to know, but without very special people I would never have graduated.

To Rich and Ann Marie Casella: I owe you a debt I cannot pay, but I do my best to make you proud every day. I love and appreciate you more than words can ever express.

To Jack Wiltshire for stepping in with answers when I had a lifetime of questions. Your warmth, guidance, and faith in me kept me going.

To Charles Leighton whose patience, wisdom and brilliance taught me everything I needed to know about myself.

To Michele and Mike Hartigan, who always support my latest endeavors but, more important, also share their greatest accomplishments (Sean and Kyle) with me whenever I need an oxytocin hit.

To Sean and Kyle Hartigan, for teaching me what it means to be an aunt. You have kept me going in the face of more challenges than you will ever know.

To Jennie and Andrew Goodman: in addition to blessing me with a beautiful iPad on which I wrote most of this book, you have kept your front-row tickets to watch my life unfold in ways I can barely understand some days. Through it all, you are the sister and brother who have given my life an anchor and sense of belonging. You guys mean everything to me.

To Dr's. Glenn & Christine Foss, God smiled on me the day our paths crossed so many years ago. As two of the main pillars in my life, I always know where to stand when the storms hit. Thank you for sharing your warmth, love, insight, wisdom, and spirit. Your love, support and friendship seem to have no limits.

To Giselle Foss: thank you for sitting and listening to my thoughts on this topic long before it evolved into a book. Your interest and enthusiasm let me know that all ages could benefit from this teaching.

To Lisa Settineri Hlifka: your energy is contagious but so is your love, support, understanding and loyalty. We have come a long way, I can't wait to see what the next 50 years bring.

To Uncle Milton and Aunt Rose, for showing the rest of us, that life isn't always fun so you'd better make your own. You have redefined "Happy Hour"

To Tom Gardner, you have known what I should be doing with my life and have never stopped pushing me towards it. Every friend should have your instincts and patience. You are a gift.

To Pat Fernot: you have impeccable timing. You always seem to know what I need and when I need it. You exemplify the meaning of friendship.

To all of the kids who have shared their lives with me in order to find their path. You have kept me on mine. You will each live in my heart forever.

To Hank Decker, for reminding me once again that a little love can change a life. Thank you for the front row seat.

To Anthony Bolognini: your gifted hands helped me to survive these endless hours at my desk. You have a special gift, my friend. I'm so happy that you are still in my life.

Barbara Minch, you have never failed to believe in me; on so many levels, you are my biggest fan—and I am yours.

To the myriad of friends I am blessed to have in my life: you are my family through it all. You have listened to my ideas, my latest epiphanies, and my brainstorms, and you never doubted that something great would come from all my effort. You are my family.

To the Scappaturas: some friends are just meant to be family. I love all of you!

To my mom, who went from patiently listening to my latest discoveries and perceptions to understanding them right along with me. I know my thirst to understand human behavior comes from you. And to my dad: thank you for showing me what strength, discipline, and loyalty can mean in a life and how to "improvise" when I'm stuck.

Thanks to all of the brilliant, scientific minds that found a way to bring the neuroscience world a little closer to the rest of us.

Made in the USA
Charleston, SC
24 May 2015